The Basics Of Psychedelic Medicine

Ewan .I Savage

All rights reserved. Copyright © 2023 Ewan .I Savage

COPYRIGHT © 2023 Ewan .I Savage

All rights reserved.

No part of this book must be reproduced, stored in a retrieval system, or shared by any means, electronic, mechanical, photocopying, recording, or otherwise, without written permission from the publisher.

Every precaution has been taken in the preparation of this book; still the publisher and author assume no responsibility for errors or omissions. Nor do they assume any liability for damages resulting from the use of the information contained herein.

Legal Notice:

This book is copyright protected and is only meant for your individual use. You are not allowed to amend, distribute, sell, use, quote or paraphrase any of its part without the written consent of the author or publisher.

Introduction

This is a comprehensive exploration of the world of psychedelics and their potential benefits. It delves into various aspects of psychedelics, providing a wealth of information for beginners and those interested in exploring the therapeutic and consciousness-expanding properties of these substances.

The book begins by sharing personal experiences of individuals who have found healing and transformation through psychedelics. These stories illustrate how psychedelics can be used to process grief, heal trauma, gain empathy, reignite spirituality, and even enhance the parent-child connection.

"Psychedelics 101" serves as an introductory chapter, offering readers a foundational understanding of psychedelics. It covers the basics of psychedelics, their history, and their potential therapeutic uses. Additionally, it provides an overview of psychedelic therapy, integration, and microdosing.

The book explores the origins of psychedelics in religious and spiritual practices, shedding light on their historical significance. It also addresses sensitive topics such as sexual abuse in psychedelic ceremonies and the legal status of these substances under the Controlled Substances Act.

Individual psychedelics, such as ketamine, psilocybin mushrooms, ayahuasca, MDMA, LSD, San Pedro, ibogaine, and DMT, are discussed in dedicated chapters. Each chapter provides a beginner's guide to the respective psychedelic, its effects, potential therapeutic applications, and harm reduction strategies.

For those interested in exploring ketamine therapy, the book offers insights into its use for treatment-resistant depression and suicidal ideation. It also discusses ketamine-assisted psychotherapy and at-home, sublingual ketamine study results.

Readers seeking information on other psychedelics will find valuable guidance on topics such as microdosing, finding ayahuasca retreats, MDMA's potential in treating PTSD, LSD microdosing, the significance of San Pedro, sustainability concerns with peyote, and the use of ibogaine for substance dependency.

The book addresses safety and responsible use throughout, emphasizing harm reduction strategies and the importance of informed, intentional psychedelic experiences.

In summary, this book provides a comprehensive and accessible resource for those interested in the therapeutic and transformative potential of psychedelics. It covers a wide range of psychedelics and their applications, making it a valuable guide for beginners and anyone looking to explore these powerful medicines.

Contents

PART ONE	1
PROCESSING GRIEF	2
HEALING TRAUMA	8
GAINING EMPATHY	11
REIGNITING SPIRITUALITY	13
CONNECTING WITH MY CHILD	16
PART TWO	19
A BEGINNER'S GUIDE TO PSYCHEDELICS	20
A BEGINNER'S GUIDE TO PSYCHEDELIC THERAPY	34
A BEGINNER'S GUIDE TO PSYCHEDELIC INTEGRATION	49
A BEGINNER'S GUIDE TO MICRODOSING	59
WHERE DO I START?	71
PSYCHEDELICS AND RELIGIOUS ORIGINS	81
SEXUAL ABUSE IN PSYCHEDELIC CEREMONIES	89
PSYCHEDELICS AND THE CONTROLLED SUBSTANCES ACT	103
PSYCHEDELIC HARM REDUCTION STRATEGIES AND STUDIES	109
PART THREEKETAMINE	115
A BEGINNER'S GUIDE TO KETAMINE	117
AT-HOME, SUBLINGUAL KETAMINE STUDY RESULTS	132
KETAMINE AND TREATMENT-RESISTANT DEPRESSION	151
CAN KETAMINE THERAPY HELP WITH SUICIDAL IDEATION?	160
KETAMINE ASSISTED PSYCHOTHERAPY	166
PART FOUR	174
A BEGINNER'S GUIDE TO PSILOCYBIN	175

HOW TO MICRODOSE WITH PSILOCYBIN MUSHROOMS	184
PART FIVE AYAHUASCA	192
A BEGINNER'S GUIDE TO AYAHUASCA	193
FINDING YOUR AYAHUASCA RETREAT	205
PART SIX MDMA	215
A BEGINNER'S GUIDE TO MDMA	216
MDMA AND PTSD	227
PART SEVEN LSD	236
A BEGINNER'S GUIDE TO LSD	237
GUIDE TO MICRODOSING LSD	247
PART EIGHT	252
A BEGINNER'S GUIDE TO SAN PEDRO	253
WHY PEYOTE SUSTAINABILITY MATTERS	270
PEYOTE LEGALITY AND RELIGIOUS FREEDOM FOR SETTLERS	280
PART NINE IBOGAINE	289
A BEGINNER'S GUIDE TO IBOGAINE	290
IBOGAINE FOR SUBSTANCE DEPENDENCY	305
PART TEN	322
A BEGINNER'S GUIDE TO DMT	323
A BEGINNER'S GUIDE TO 5-MEO-DMT	334

PART ONE
FIVE PERSONAL EXPERIENCES

"I understood that our entire universe is contained in the mind and the spirit. We may choose not to find access to it, we may even deny its existence, but it is indeed there inside us, and there are chemicals that can catalyze its availability."

Alexander Shulgin

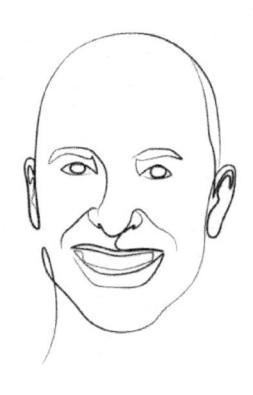

ONE
PROCESSING GRIEF
MATT ZEMON, MSC

NOVEMBER 1971

Two weeks ago you were conceived. Your father's complexities and mine have merged, come together to make a wholly different person--you. Already I have signs that you are within me, growing, struggling for life, becoming whole. I am so proud and so pleased to be nurturing you and sheltering you, although I still find it all overwhelming and almost unbelievable. All miracles are almost unbelievable to us. The creation of life is so awe-inspiring; so incomprehensible. For you will not only be (I pray) a healthy little pink body with ten toes and ten fingers and eyelashes as delicate as breath, you will also be a mind. A soul. A heart, A person as intricate, as unique, as unpredictable as any stranger. And yet you are mine.

I want to tell you, my darling, that I love you. I didn't start loving you today, or two weeks ago. I have loved you for many, many years; I don't know if other people feel that way too. I only know that as a girl, I already loved my unborn children with a devotion and a sincerity that I've never known for anyone else. I've thought so often of you, my firstborn. For the last several months, I've been praying for you to happen soon. You are very, very wanted. You are in no way an accident. I've known you, yearning for you, been anxious to hold you, for at least half my life.

I'm not afraid for you, though I suppose I should be. The dangers of the world outside our door are tremendous, and frightening. The complexities are staggering. The problems sometimes seem hopeless. Will you have fresh air to breathe, will you be allowed to develop in a world of peace, will the birds still be singing when you are an adult? The dangers inside our door are even more terrifying. I do not know what is going to happen to my marriage, and whatever happens will certainly affect you and your happiness. I'm sorry I can make no promises about anything. I would like to be able to promise you at least health and happiness, if not fortune.

But whatever happens, I can't be afraid. I have faith in us, you see. And in God. And strange, I trust you. I trust that you will be one of the finest people God ever made. I trust that you will find your way, and that it will be a good way. I hope so that I can help you, and that I don't hinder you too much.

I know you will be a very special kind of person. That sounds terribly conceited, but it really isn't. I want to try so hard to help you love life. And not to hate. I don't know if I can do that or not. Perhaps you'll have to do it all by yourself.

You will probably never really know me, nor I you. And that seems a terrible pity, but it is the way of the world. Parents and children rarely know or are able to see each other as people. I will forever be Your Mother, you will forever be My Child. Perhaps we will grow together; if we're lucky we will understand each other somewhat. Perhaps some of our values will be the same; some of our ideas and hopes shared in common.

But you will live in a different world entirely, I will try to give you all I can, but it can never ever be enough. You'll still skin your knees and be rejected by some playmates. Someday you'll fail at something you want very badly to succeed in. Someday you'll lose someone you love very much. There will be times when you doubt everything about your life, yourself, the things you've been taught, your very worth as a human being.

I hope you never doubt God. Because faith will help you. And for whatever comfort it may be at any time in your life, know that I love you dearly. Know that I believe in you. My tiny son or daughter, you have hardly begun your existence. Yet I believe that someday you will do great things. Like make someone else happy. Like be generous when it's hard to be. Like forgive when revenge would be sweet indeed. I believe you can be, and will be, strong and loving. I hope you will make the world a better place for all of us. But whatever you do, or become--whatever you are--I'm very glad you are mine.

-Rosemary Zemon, age 25

APRIL 25, 1995

I was 22 when my mom died. She was just 49.

I had experienced death before--my grandmother, great aunt... even my dad. It wasn't the same.

When my mom died, it felt like a piece of my heart was ripped out of me. I could feel the emptiness.

When we buried her, I wailed.

I didn't know what it meant to wail before that day. That day I unleashed a primal scream into the world. I cried so hard I couldn't breathe. I sobbed impossibly large tears. That day I wailed, and I discovered what the low side of my emotional range was.

That day I lost any faith I had in God.

And then life moved on, as it does.

I worked and missed my mom.

I got married and missed my mom.

I had kids and missed my mom.

I put this part of me into a drawer and just went on with living, as the living do.

And life was fine.

Twenty-four years later, I would reconnect with my mom through a guided psilocybin experience.

APRIL 25, 2019

I went into my psychedelic mushroom journey with no real expectations. I was never a drug person. I had tried pot several times and decided it wasn't for me. I didn't even drink that much. In retrospect, I clearly had control issues and felt more comfortable when I maintained the perception of being in control.

Some good friends suggested that I try a guided psilocybin experience. I didn't even know what psilocybin was or why I would want to try it. They talked about how much people learned through these experiences. I liked learning. They talked about it being like going on a trip in your mind. I liked to travel, so I agreed and surrendered to the opportunity.

Our guide told us we would be safe. He prepared us for the potential of a challenging experience and said that if that happened, to ask whatever was causing fear or anxiety what it wanted to teach us. He asked us to bring something important to us from our childhood to the ceremony. I brought the letter that my mom wrote to me while she was pregnant.

He built an altar. We brought up our mementos. We meditated. We ate the mushrooms. We meditated some more.

And then I was gone.

Gone.

I had melted into the ground and was watching and feeling the world breathe.

In waves, I became aware of my grandparents, great-grandparents, and all of the people I was connected to in this world.

I felt connected to the earth, trees, and sky in a way I had never felt before.

And I felt loved.

Unconditionally loved.

And I realized I was safe.

And I realized I didn't remember what it felt like to truly feel loved and safe. Ever.

Ever.

And I realized that because I didn't remember what it felt like to truly feel loved, I hadn't been able to truly share love. With my wife. With my kids. With my sister. With my friends. With the world.

I had been living my life scared.

I was scared of dying.

And then I saw my mom. And felt her. And I instantly understood that she wasn't gone; she was a part of me. And I was carrying her essence forward.

I could pull a string from her to me. And then through me to my kids. We were all connected. We were all carrying each other.

And I felt this in my heart.

I viscerally felt that I was connected to her and that we were united. That we had always been united and would always be united. The hole in my heart was, for the first time in 24 years, full.

And in that instant, I realized my perception of God was wrong. I could see a world that was bigger than anything I had ever conceived. I could feel a connectedness that spanned time and space. I could understand in my soul that we are all part of something bigger. I could understand the truth that we are all brothers and sisters.

And I remembered joy. True joy.

And I was no longer scared.

And I was no longer afraid of dying.

And I knew that I was loved.

And I knew that I was safe.
And always had been.
And always will be.

TWO
HEALING TRAUMA
MATT ZEMON, MSC

When I was going through puberty I had inappropriate, intimate contact with an extended family member who was more than a decade older than me. The physical contact had started a few years before and progressed. The last time it happened, I remember snapping into an awareness of how wrong this situation was and being mortified. The experience went from feeling good to feeling awful in a flash.

For years I felt guilt. If I was honest with myself, I had liked the feeling of touching her. I had enjoyed the feeling of being touched. I felt that this situation was my fault. That my raging hormones drove this, that I should have known better.

Over time I learned to understand that the adult is the one that is responsible for establishing and maintaining boundaries. That my physiological responses were normal and that the requests made of me were simply not appropriate. But I didn't know that then, and that knowledge didn't take away the feelings associated with the experience.

Eventually, I disconnected contact with her and cut her out of my life. That felt good and empowering. But while those actions removed the reminder, they didn't heal anything. My attempt to compartmentalize this part of my life left me with a festering open wound. A wound that leaked shame. A wound that oozed guilt.

This was a part of my life that I couldn't talk to anyone about. I moved forward and pretended it didn't happen. But it did happen. And I knew it did.

While, for the most part, I didn't think about her or it, every now and then, I would be reminded, and I would feel my ears getting red, and a pit in my stomach would come back as my body reminded me of my childhood trauma.

It had been more than 25 years since I had last seen her when she came to me during a psychedelic experience. To be clear, this was not related to the intention I had set for this journey, nor was it something I had asked to be healed from. After all this time, it was an unexpected shock to find myself looking at her again, watching the experience unfold in front of me like I was an observer in someone else's life.

Watching this iteration, there was no shame or guilt. This time, when I looked at her, I saw something different than the misguided perpetrator I had constructed. This time I saw her as sad. Lonely. Helpless. Scared.

Without condoning or forgiving her actions, I could see her as a human being that was hurt. Who had been effectively abandoned by her father. Who was not as pretty, smart, or talented as her sibling. A human who was having a hard time moderating her drug and alcohol use. A human who was looking anywhere and everywhere for love and not finding it.

Without condoning or forgiving her actions, I could understand her feelings of insecurity.

Without condoning or forgiving her actions, I had genuine empathy for her.

And with genuine empathy firmly established, I felt my wounds close.

At this moment, the psychedelic medicine allowed me to disassociate from myself, re-look at an experience that had haunted me for years, and release the anger, hatred, embarrassment, guilt, and shame that had weighed me down for decades without me even realizing it.

THREE
GAINING EMPATHY
MATT ZEMON, MSC

My daughter is smart. Funny. Creative.
My daughter is loving. Generous. Kind.
My daughter is not neurotypical.

I didn't even know what this was or meant. My wife and I knew that she was different; we just didn't have any context in which to understand her. When she was little, she devoured books and understood plot lines well beyond her years. We just assumed she was really smart.

In middle school, her social differences became more apparent, and we started to understand that she didn't see or process social cues the same way we did.

And then the panic attacks began. We would find her curled up in a ball on the stairs or in the hallway, inconsolably crying. And we didn't know what to do.

Between a gifted therapist and dialectical behavior therapy (DBT) training, she learned healthy ways to cope with stress and regulate emotions while becoming more successful in social situations. We learned the theory behind some of her processing differences and practical tactics for how to co-exist and foster independence.

And while I could understand the theory and loved her very much, I didn't feel like I could understand what she was experiencing or in any way relate to what her way of living in the world felt like.

During an ayahuasca ceremony, I found myself sitting next to her in an amusement park car as we entered some kind of carnival funhouse. For the most part, everything in this funhouse was just a little off. A little creepy. A little scary. Every now and then we would turn a corner and something would happen that was very scary. My heart rate would increase, and I would feel like I wanted to scream. Then, as quickly as the terrifying part happened, the ride would return to just a baseline level of discomfort.

It was in this psychedelic-induced funhouse that, for the first time, I started to understand what it might feel like to experience a world that was different than the safe, optimistic, abundant one that I live in. To have an overwhelming desire to put on headphones to tune out sounds that are causing me agitation. To take a break from the creepy ride and get completely absorbed in the making of a piece of art. To decide to create my own worlds the way I want them to be through intense rounds of dungeons and dragons.

My daughter is amazing. She has a gift of sight that allows her not just to see the characters she creates but to truly see her friends. Psychedelic medicine empowered me to emotionally understand her in ways that years of theoretical training did not.

FOUR
REIGNITING SPIRITUALITY
MATT ZEMON, MSC

My mother was Catholic and my father was Jewish. At dinner parties I used to say I was a Cashew. The reality is I didn't have a strong belief system at all.

Early on, I couldn't understand how Christian friends would say my grandmother wasn't going to heaven because she was Jewish. That didn't feel right. At the same time, I couldn't understand how the Jewish people were the chosen ones and what that meant to the Christian people. Or the Muslims. Or Hindus. Or….

My mind couldn't conceive of a heaven or hell; the idea of a place where our souls would gather after our time on earth just didn't make sense to me.

Then came my experience with 5-MeO-DMT, commonly known as Bufo.

Before I get there, let me step back a bit.

In psychedelic experience after psychedelic experience, I have felt more love than I knew was possible. After my mom died, I had felt and learned the low end of my emotional range, but I didn't know how high my upper range could go.

In these psychedelic experiences, I felt like there was infinite time and abundance. That there was pure bliss. That there was beauty in what used to look ordinary. That we are all connected. That we are all beings of love.

These experiences taught me to take a bigger view. To not think in terms of "world" but rather in terms of "universe." To not think of "lifetimes" but in terms of "millions of years." To not think not of "my nuclear family" but of all of us as "one collective family."

Within seconds of inhaling 5-MeO-DMT I saw myself melting into a pyramid of silver liquid and then literally became nothing but energy. My body and I were completely gone. Around me there was a loud Om. More specifically, a loud Awwwww….ooooooooh…..mmmmm which later I learned is the primal, cosmic sound of the source in many traditions.

I could feel the energy and the vibrations around me. Everything and everyone was pure energy.

And it was beautiful. A euphoria in this zone of existence was well beyond anything I had ever experienced or imagined.

There was absolutely no fear. No fear of dying. No fear of not being enough. I was more alive than I ever was before and yet there was no me.

After being a part of the vibrations of the universe, I started to recognize again that there was a me and a body. The vibrations felt wonderful, but now I could feel the energy inside of me radiating out. I could point my fingers toward each other and feel the energy connect between them. I could put my hand over my heart and stomach and feel the energy in those regions.

I was taking deep, cosmic breaths Sucking in the energy. Exhaling the energy.

I could swim in it.

I wept tears of joy. Tears of connection.

I knew I was powerful. Good. Deserving of love. That I was love.

There was no sense of time, but my understanding is this entire journey was about 20 minutes.

I had never prayed as deeply as I did that day. Ever.

I had never felt more connected to the power of the universe.

I had never felt as happy in my life.

I emerged with a strong belief in God.

I emerged able to comprehend the idea of a place that has room for everyone, that is safe and loving. That is paradise. That is heaven.

FIVE
CONNECTING WITH MY CHILD
MATT ZEMON, MSC

What would you do if your 16-year-old child asked to watch you do drugs?

Cole is a smart and sensitive agender kid who has been vocal with us that he does not experiment with drugs or alcohol, so I was surprised (shocked) when they asked if they could go on a psychedelic retreat with me. I asked them if they wanted to try psychedelics, and they said they did not; they just wanted to learn more about what I was working on. This seemed like a reasonable request. At the same time, I wondered if I would be able to give myself over to the medicine completely in front of them. This was a level of "letting go" that I had not contemplated before.

This particular psychedelic retreat had 22 participants and started with three days of preparation. During this period there were 10-12 hours a day of lectures on consciousness, group discussions, and meditations. People shared personal stories about their struggles, their relationships, their insecurities, and their traumas.

On the fourth day, we each took the "sacramental meditation" and made ourselves comfortable throughout the beautiful property where the retreat was located. Cole was enlisted as one of the assistants, ensuring everyone stayed hydrated during journeys that lasted about six hours, guiding people to the restrooms, and delivering blankets as needed.

As we each dropped into our psychedelic experiences, Cole watched the transformations take place. While they couldn't know precisely what was happening in anyone's mind, they could see that some people were amazed at what they were seeing, others were feeling enormous waves of love, and some were working through challenging experiences.

At one point, Cole came and checked on me. I was deep into my journey, but when they appeared they immediately snapped into focus. I hugged Cole tightly, and I could visualize my blood and their blood combining and wrapping around us. I could see our DNA intertwining. During that embrace, I told them that I lost both of my parents when I was too young and that no one gives an instruction manual on how to be a parent. I told them that I was doing the best that I knew how to do and that I wanted them to know that I loved them very much.

We stayed embraced for a while longer, then they moved on to help others, and I continued with my journey.

That evening we gathered in the large living room of the retreat leader's house. A fire crackled in the fireplace, and everyone was exhausted from a long day of "traveling." Cole and I were lying on an oversized beanbag chair next to each other. One by one, people shared what they had experienced. Cole watched as grown men cried and held each other. Cole listened as adults talked about past hurts, marriage challenges, fears, and regrets and how the psychedelic medicine helped them reframe. Cole heard people talk about how much love and safety they felt when experiencing the psychedelic medicine and how, through the medicine, they were able to examine aspects of their life without the usual shame and guilt that accompanied it.

As Cole and I lay there, I couldn't help but think that I had never had an experience like this when I was their age. When I was 16, I looked at adults as grown-ups who had life figured out. I didn't realize that adults struggled with issues of acceptance, purpose, love, and forgiveness. I didn't imagine that adults would still have relationship issues with their parents that they would still be working out. I didn't understand that adults still might not know what they want to do when they grew up. I didn't think that things that had happened to adults while they were kids would still cause tremendous pain decades later.

The next day was the integration day. During a time of sharing, Cole thanked the group for the support they had given me. Cole said they could see the difference this work was making in me and our family and that I had never been more "emotionally available." I didn't have Cole's vocabulary when I was their age, nor did I have their understanding of human interconnectedness. I would not have used the expression "emotionally available," nor would I have had the depth to understand what it meant.

It was hard to let go and be completely vulnerable in front of my child, yet I am grateful to have been able to share this experience with them. I am glad they had the opportunity to see me in a raw emotional state and that we could share a moment of deep connectedness. I am grateful that I could put them in a situation where they could see adults as humans, processing their real emotions. My hope is that through this experience, Cole understands sooner than I did how important it is to align actions with purpose and that no amount of material things will bring happiness.

I walked away from this retreat with a deeper appreciation of Cole as another fellow human. While I am their father, Cole is their own person on their own path. I am grateful that our lives have crossed and that I have the privilege to watch them grow. And I recognize that just like at this retreat, while we are embraced for a moment in time, Cole will move on with their journey.

My hope is that Cole looks back at this experience and remembers that they were, and are, loved deeply.

PART TWO
PSYCHEDELICS 101

"Psychedelics (will) be for psychiatry what the microscope is for biology or the telescope is for astronomy. These tools make it possible to study important processes that under normal circumstances are not available for direct observation."

Dr. Stanislav Grof, MD

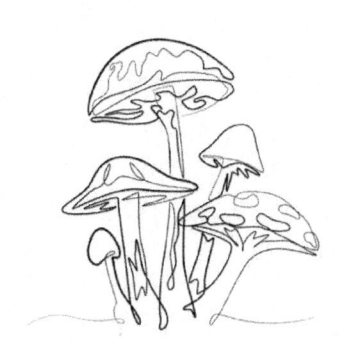

SIX
A BEGINNER'S GUIDE TO PSYCHEDELICS
LEIA FRIEDWOMAN, MS

MEDICALLY REVIEWED BY DR. DAVID COX, PHD, ABPP

Psychedelics, sometimes referred to as hallucinogens or entheogen, are a group of substances that can lead to an altered state of consciousness. Some well-known examples include psilocybin containing mushrooms, LSD (acid), dimethyl-tryptamine (DMT), and mescaline which is found in the San Pedro and peyote cactus. The word psychedelic derives from the Greek *psyche*, meaning mind, and *delos*, meaning manifesting.

Humphrey Osmond, a British psychiatrist, coined the term "psychedelic" in the 1950s after he discovered that LSD helped patients with alcoholism (Dyck, 2006). The results of the LSD treatment far surpassed any other interventions available at the time. Osmond did not discover LSD; it was first synthesized by a Swiss chemist named Albert Hofmann in the 1930s. April 19th, 1943, also known as "bicycle day," is the anniversary of the world's first acid trip, a holiday that is still celebrated by some psychedelic enthusiasts today. Osmond later introduced famous poet and author Aldous Huxley to mescaline; the experiences had such a profound effect that it led Huxley to write *The Doors of Perception*.

In 1955, a banker named R. Gordon Wasson who was interested in mushrooms traveled to Oaxaca, Mexico and met Maria Sabina, a Mazatec shaman. She introduced him to the sacred psilocybe mushrooms that grow in that area, which she used to help heal sick people in her village. Although Sabina asked Wasson not to share his experience with the mushroom, he shared it in an article for *Life Magazine (Wasson, 1959)*.

This deceit marked the introduction of psychedelic mushrooms into western society and, ultimately, a tragedy for Maria Sabina. The psychedelic tourism that the magazine article spawned permanently changed the town of Huautla, where she lived; major disagreements took place, which ultimately led to Maria Sabina's house being burned down. She moved to the outskirts of town and eventually passed away in poverty.

By the 1960s, psychedelic use was becoming more and more widespread. Commonly associated with hippie counter-culture, psychedelics probably played a role in the collective resistance to war and oppression that swelled during this era.

While these drugs are often used for recreational purposes, they also have a long history of religious and spiritual use. Indigenous cultures of present-day Peru, Columbia, Ecuador, and Brazil may have used ayahuasca for centuries. Psychedelics such as iboga can be found in African traditional medicine, where they are used to treat mental illness and physical ailments. Psychedelic substances can be found on all continents except Antarctica, so it's safe to assume that wherever there is history of human civilization, psychedelics have played some role in medicinal or spiritual use.

Psychedelics are currently being examined for their potential to improve quality of life by treating mental illnesses such as depression, anxiety, obsessive-compulsive disorder, addiction, PTSD, eating disorders, and easing anxiety for patients with a terminal illnesses (Grob et al., 2011; Krediet et al., 2020; Moreno, Wiegand, Taitano, & Delgado, 2006; Muttoni, Ardissino, & John, 2019; Roseman, Nutt, & Carhart-Harris, 2018; Tófoli & de Araujo,

2016). Researchers have also found that psychedelics can increase creativity, improve mood, and more (Baggott, 2015; Fadiman & Korb, 2019).

The following sections contain common concerns and questions asked by people who are interested in taking psychedelics.

ARE PSYCHEDELIC DRUGS ADDICTIVE?

Addiction is a complex term. This chapter offers an evidence-based perspective on addiction, informed by the Psychedelic Harm Reduction and Integration model (PHRI), a transtheoretical and transdiagnostic clinical approach to working with patients who are using or considering using psychedelics in any context (Gorman, Nielson, Molinar, Cassidy, & Sabbagh, 2021). According to the authors, "PHRI represents a shift away from assessment limited to untoward outcomes of psychedelic use and abstinence-based addiction treatment paradigms and toward a stance of compassionate, destigmatizing acceptance of patients' choices."

This approach contrasts to the standard clinical understanding of addiction provided by The Diagnostic and Statistical Manual of mental disorders (DSM-5). The DSM-5 uses the name Substance Use Disorder for what is commonly referred to as addiction. If a person is unable to stop consuming a substance despite wanting to, and if the use of a substance causes significant problems in someone's life, they may have substance use disorder. The DSM-5 lists 11 symptoms that indicate that substance use disorder may be present. Depending on the number of criteria that a person meets, they will be diagnosed as having mild, moderate, or severe substance use disorder. Only a licensed professional can diagnose someone with a mental illness.

In terms of developing physical dependence, classic, serotonergic psychedelics are not addictive. Specifically, people do not crave them after use due to physiological dependence, and physiological withdrawal symptoms do not occur after ingesting psychedelics, even after multiple psychedelic experiences.

Ketamine might have the highest potential for abuse among the more popular psychedelics today, although, as of the date of this publication, there are no case reports of addiction arising from therapeutic use. Due to the short duration of action (around one to three hours), ketamine can be used regularly without monopolizing most of a person's waking hours like taking LSD daily would. Case reports from daily users indicate that some people have struggled with a marker of a substance use disorder, such as unsuccessful attempts to control the use or quit, despite long-term negative consequences to one's health. Prolonged ketamine overuse is associated with major health issues, including kidney, bladder, and heart issues, cognitive issues, and decreased sociability. Over time, daily ketamine users can develop a lasting tolerance to the substance, requiring higher doses to reach the desired effect. This is another marker of addiction: using increasingly larger amounts of the substance or using it for longer than intended.

From the perspective that addiction is a problematic relationship to something that drives the user to seek it out for consumption despite negative consequences, psychedelics could be addictive for some people.

Due to rapidly built physical tolerance, daily use is a challenge for classic psychedelics such as LSD and psilocybin mushrooms. Increasing one's psychedelic dose significantly and/or taking a break of 2-3 days is the only effective way for one's psychedelic use to have any discernible effect after a period of daily dosing. Even in the case of microdosing, people typically have two or more rest days each week on which they do not take the sub-perceptual dose of the psychedelic.

Psychologically, the introspective nature of psychedelics allows some people to intuit if they are using the drug too much or not enough.

Although most people do not take high doses every day, psychedelics can certainly be used as a crutch. For example, some people find that microdosing helps them access a level of creativity, energy, or mood that they lack in their normal day-to-day lives. In the absence of microdosing, the person cannot perform at the optimum level that they want to. This may lead to what some would regard as a dependent relationship. Another example would be a person attending repeated ayahuasca ceremonies without doing meaningful integration work or implementing change in their life based on what the journeys revealed.

Spiritual bypassing is using spiritual concepts, lingo, and phenomena to excuse oneself from doing the emotional, psychological, developmental, and relational work to actually address core issues. The late John Welwood coined the term "spiritual bypassing" in his book, *Toward a Psychology of Awakening.* While he doesn't touch on psychedelics directly in the book, psychedelic use can become a form of spiritual bypassing, whereby the person goes back repeatedly into the psychedelic state without working on their issues outside of the psychedelic journey and without integrating the insights into their daily life.

Chögyam Trungpa said it well: "Ego is able to convert anything to its own use, even spirituality."

Bottom line: Whether a person is addicted to psychedelics would have to be established by a licensed clinician who is familiar with the psychedelic terrain. If you're feeling concerned about your relationship to psychedelics, assess how many of these criteria apply to you and consider seeking out help from peer and/or professional support person(s), especially those who practice with the PHRI.

While psychedelics can instigate profound healing experiences, they can also bring about difficult, frightening, confusing, and painful experiences. As a result, it is important to have appropriate support following a journey. A trained therapist can help a person integrate challenging experiences from the trip into their daily life and path toward healing. In addition, supportive community groups can provide ongoing guidance and assistance. By offering both professional and peer support, these resources can help ensure that psychedelics are used safely and effectively to promote healing and growth.

Psychedelics do not have to be focused solely on mental health or any sort of self-improvement; they can be used purely for pleasure, as well. From a cognitive liberty perspective, the right to alter one's own consciousness belongs to each person.

SIDE EFFECTS OF PSYCHEDELIC DRUGS

The side effects of psychedelic drugs vary depending on the substance, dose, set, and setting of the person taking them.

Dosage means how much of the psychedelic is consumed. Psychedelics can have vastly different effects, solely depending on the dosage. *Set* can be thought of as the inner setting of the person; their mental, physical, and emotional state. The intention (or expectation) for the use of the psychedelic can also be part of the person's set. *Setting* is where the person is for the experience. Being alone versus being with people is an aspect of the setting, as is the type and level of sensory stimulation.

The most common side effects of psychedelics are shifts in mood, visual hallucinations, sensory changes (including sensitivity), an altered perception of time, and differences in thought and perspective from what is typical for the person.

Psychedelics also produce physical side effects, including changes in heart rate, blood pressure, and body temperature. People may experience weakness, lack of coordination, dizziness, and/or shaking. Nausea, diarrhea, and vomiting are also possible (especially with ayahuasca, ibogaine, and sometimes psilocybin mushrooms).

Research has documented that some people have mystical experiences when they take a psychedelic, especially in higher doses (Winkelman, 2017). Reports have also indicated that subject to the context in which they take the psychedelic, nature-relatedness can increase with psychedelic use (Kettner, Gandy, Haijen, & Carhart-Harris, 2019).

Psychedelics are great for exploring the depths of your psyche, but they can also bring up difficult material. You might find yourself feeling intense and even unsafe during these shifts in mood - having a supportive person around makes all the difference!

LEGAL STATUS OF PSYCHEDELIC DRUGS

"Psychedelics are illegal not because a loving government is concerned that you may jump out of a third-story window. Psychedelics are illegal because they dissolve opinion structures and culturally laid down models of behavior and information processing. They open you up to the possibility that everything you know is wrong."

Terrence McKenna, ethnobotanist and mystic

Ketamine is currently the only legal psychedelic widely available in America.

When the Controlled Substances Act was passed in 1970, it effectively criminalized the use of psychedelics in the United States. While some advocate for this law on the grounds of public health, the truth is that it was motivated by racism and pro-war sentiments. The passage of the Controlled Substances Act was a way to quash dissent and enforce conformity. Psychedelics were seen as a way to "expand consciousness" and challenge authority, making them a threat to those in power. As a result, they were outlawed in an effort to maintain the status quo.

Author Dan Baum was working on a book in 1994 when he sought out Jonathan Ehrlichman, Nixon's domestic-policy adviser, and a co-conspirator in the Watergate Scandal, to ask some questions about the politics of drug prohibition.

In his report *Legalize It All: How to Win the War on Drugs (Baum, 2016)*, Baum states:

I started to ask Ehrlichman a series of earnest, wonky questions that he impatiently waved away. "You want to know what this was really all about?" he asked with the bluntness of a man who, after public disgrace and a stretch in federal prison, had little left to protect. "The Nixon campaign in 1968, and the Nixon White House after that, had two enemies: the antiwar left and black people. You understand what I'm saying? We knew we couldn't make it illegal to be either against the war or black, but by getting the public to associate the hippies with marijuana and blacks with heroin, and then criminalizing both heavily, we could disrupt those communities. We could arrest their leaders, raid their homes, break up their meetings, and vilify them night after night on the evening news. Did we know we were lying about the drugs? Of course we did."

Although Nixon initiated this political move, no president since has attempted to dismantle it. The drug war is used as an excuse to invade and dismantle sovereign nations and promotes the militarization of the police. Meanwhile, billions of dollars have been wasted on a war on drugs, or more accurately, a war on drug users, especially black and brown people, as well as poor people.

Baum goes on to say, "the desire for altered states of consciousness creates a market, and in suppressing that market we have created a class of genuine bad guys — pushers, gangbangers, smugglers, killers. Addiction is a hideous condition, but it's rare. Most of what we hate and fear about drugs — the violence, the overdoses, the criminality — derives from prohibition, not drugs."

DECRIMINALIZATION: IS IT HELPFUL?

Portugal is a great example of how decriminalizing drugs can actually be beneficial for public health (Gonçalves, Lourenço, & Silva, 2015; Mendes, Pacheco, Nunes, Crespo, & Cruz, 2019). After decriminalization, more people sought out treatment for substance dependence, drug-related deaths such as overdose declined, disease transmission and incarceration numbers dropped, rates of marijuana use went up, and rates of opioid use went down. Fewer resources go toward policing, incarceration, and medical costs associated with overdose. As a result, there are more resources available for harm reduction services, such as education and treatment for substance dependence.

In the 2020 election, the state of Oregon voted to decriminalize all drugs, including heroin, cocaine, methamphetamine, MDMA, psilocybin mushrooms, LSD, and more. The results after the first year showed a 60% decrease in the number of people arrested for any drug offense (3,700 vs. 9,100) and that 16,000 people have accessed support services. There is expected improvement as more services and education are rolled out. Oregon also legalized psilocybin for therapeutic use in a licensed and regulated environment. Several cities have decriminalized naturally occurring psychedelics, and more are expected to do the same.

Oakland, CA, was the first jurisdiction to decriminalize nature. The term "decriminalization" is a bit of a misnomer. The local government voted that possession of DMT, psilocybin mushrooms, iboga/ibogaine, and mescaline-containing cacti should be the lowest priority of law enforcement to the police. A more fitting term might be "deprioritization." The sale of these substances can still get a person in trouble for drug trafficking.

Plenty of psychedelic enthusiasts and holistic practitioners rejoiced when this monumental vote took place. Several other cities have since followed suit. However, this movement to decriminalize naturally occurring psychedelics or entheogens has received some criticism.

Peyotist Dawn Davis, PhD, criticized Decriminalize Nature for not consulting indigenous people before including peyote in a city resolution. She reached out to the Oakland City Council, recognizing that indigenous consultation and consultation with the Native American Church did not occur. Davis, in collaboration with the National Council of Native American Churches (NCNAC) and Indigenous Peyote Conservation Initiative (IPCI), released this statement about Decriminalize Nature explicitly including peyote in their brand image and messaging, and not consulting indigenous people beforehand:

"It is extremely important that peyote be preserved for utilization by and for indigenous peoples. Broken treaties in this land, the preciousness of native traditions, ecological threats to the medicine itself, and the importance of spiritual respect in its use makes peyote a tenuous plant to include explicitly in any decriminalization effort."

Peyote remains a tenuous issue in decriminalization initiatives. Another concern with the Decriminalize Nature movement is psychedelic exceptionalism. Psychedelic exceptionalism is the ideology driving some activists to advocate for legal protection for psychedelic drugs while not changing the drug laws about other substances. It's called psychedelic exceptionalism because it carries the assumption that psychedelics are less harmful, less addictive, and offer more potential benefits than other drugs; therefore, psychedelics should not be criminalized.

One issue of the psychedelic exceptionalism ideology is the focus on changing the penalties for possession and use of naturally occurring Schedule 1 psychedelic drugs, but not for other drugs. The disparity is in what public health researchers and harm-reductionists have been saying for a long time: criminalizing substance users is not an effective deterrent to drug use. Criminalization compounds harm because it drives suppliers and users underground, restricts educational resources, and even limits access to life-affirming services such as substance testing and treatment for substance dependence. The drug war also perpetuates racial disparities: black and brown people are incarcerated at much higher rates than white people for drug-related offenses.

Dr. Carl Hart, professor at Columbia University and recent author of the book *Drug Use for Grown-Ups,* often speaks out against psychedelic exceptionalism (Hart, 2022). Dr. Hart works to elevate the voices of people who use drugs. His work has helped many people to reframe what society knows about drug use by demonstrating that all kinds of people use drugs (even Dr. Hart, who came out of the closet this year as a heroin and methamphetamine user). He purports that there is no "typical" or "normal" drug use, but there *is* safe and sensible drug use. This position advocates for education and awareness around substances rather than prohibition or abstinence. Through understanding the body, the drugs, and their effects, Dr. Hart has remained a fully functional member of society as an attentive husband, father, academic, and taxpayer.

Cognitive liberty, also known as the right to mental self-determination, is the idea that each person is sovereign over their own consciousness. Some activists say that the prohibition of drugs is an infringement on cognitive liberty. "No benevolent government should forbid autonomous adults from altering their consciousness, as long as it does not infringe on the rights of others," Dr. Hart says in his book.

US President Joe Biden recently enacted the American Rescue Plan. This will provide funding for community-based substance use disorder services such as syringe exchange programs and other harm reduction interventions. Perhaps the tides are finally turning from prohibition ("just say *no*") to education ("just say *know*," as Timothy Leary said).

A NEW ERA FOR PSYCHEDELIC DRUGS

Clinical research has indicated that psychedelics are relatively safe substances when used properly. There are millions of anecdotal reports that affirm that people have found deeper awareness and empowerment to address their issues with the help of psychedelics. While these substances are not miracle cures, they can be viewed as tools that can be helpful for some people. Ultimately, it is up to each individual to decide whether or not to use psychedelics.

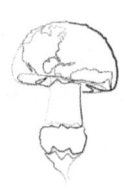

REFERENCES:

- Baggott, M. J. (2015). *Psychedelics and Creativity: a Review of the Quantitative Literature*.
- Baum, D. (2016). Legalize it All: How to Win the War on Drugs. *Harper's Magazine*.
- Dyck, E. (2006). 'Hitting Highs at Rock Bottom': LSD Treatment for Alcoholism, 1950–1970. *Social History of Medicine, 19*(2), 313-329. doi:10.1093/shm/hkl039
- Fadiman, J., & Korb, S. (2019). Might Microdosing Psychedelics Be Safe and Beneficial? An Initial Exploration. *Journal of Psychoactive Drugs, 51*(2), 118-122. doi:10.1080/02791072.2019.1593561
- Gonçalves, R., Lourenço, A., & Silva, S. N. (2015). A social cost perspective in the wake of the Portuguese strategy for

- the fight against drugs. *Int J Drug Policy, 26*(2), 199-209. doi:10.1016/j.drugpo.2014.08.017
- Gorman, I., Nielson, E. M., Molinar, A., Cassidy, K., & Sabbagh, J. (2021). Psychedelic Harm Reduction and Integration: A Transtheoretical Model for Clinical Practice. *Front Psychol, 12*, 645246. doi:10.3389/fpsyg.2021.645246
- Grob, C. S., Danforth, A. L., Chopra, G. S., Hagerty, M., McKay, C. R., Halberstadt, A. L., & Greer, G. R. (2011). Pilot Study of Psilocybin Treatment for Anxiety in Patients With Advanced-Stage Cancer. *Archives of General Psychiatry, 68*(1), 71-78. doi:10.1001/archgenpsychiatry.2010.116
- Hart, C. L. (2022). *Drug use for grown-ups: Chasing liberty in the land of fear*. Penguin.
- Kettner, H., Gandy, S., Haijen, E. C. H. M., & Carhart-Harris, R. L. (2019). From Egoism to Ecoism: Psychedelics Increase Nature Relatedness in a State-Mediated and Context-Dependent Manner. *International Journal of Environmental Research and Public Health, 16*(24), 5147. Retrieved from https://www.mdpi.com/1660-4601/16/24/5147
- Krediet, E., Bostoen, T., Breeksema, J., van Schagen, A., Passie, T., & Vermetten, E. (2020). Reviewing the Potential of Psychedelics for the Treatment of PTSD. *International Journal of Neuropsychopharmacology, 23*(6), 385-400. doi:10.1093/ijnp/pyaa018
- Mendes, R. O., Pacheco, P. G., Nunes, J., Crespo, P. S., & Cruz, M. S. (2019). Literature review on the implications of decriminalization for the care of drug users in Portugal and Brazil. *Cien Saude Colet, 24*(9), 3395-3406. doi:10.1590/1413-81232018249.27472017
- Moreno, F. A., Wiegand, C. B., Taitano, E. K., & Delgado, P. L. (2006). Safety, tolerability, and efficacy of psilocybin in 9

- patients with obsessive-compulsive disorder. *J Clin Psychiatry, 67*(11), 1735-1740. doi:10.4088/jcp.v67n1110
- Muttoni, S., Ardissino, M., & John, C. (2019). Classical psychedelics for the treatment of depression and anxiety: A systematic review. *Journal of Affective Disorders, 258*, 11-24. doi:https://doi.org/10.1016/j.jad.2019.07.076
- Roseman, L., Nutt, D. J., & Carhart-Harris, R. L. (2018). Quality of Acute Psychedelic Experience Predicts Therapeutic Efficacy of Psilocybin for Treatment-Resistant Depression. *Frontiers in pharmacology, 8*. doi:10.3389/fphar.2017.00974
- Tófoli, L. F., & de Araujo, D. B. (2016). Chapter Seven - Treating Addiction: Perspectives from EEG and Imaging Studies on Psychedelics. In N. M. Zahr & E. T. Peterson (Eds.), *International Review of Neurobiology* (Vol. 129, pp. 157-185): Academic Press.
- Wasson, R. G. (1959). Seeking the Magic Mushroom. *Life Magazine*, 42, 100-102, 104-110, 112, 114, 117-118, 120.
- Winkelman, M. J. (2017). The Mechanisms of Psychedelic Visionary Experiences: Hypotheses from Evolutionary Psychology. *Frontiers in Neuroscience, 11*. doi:10.3389/fnins.2017.00539

SEVEN

A BEGINNER'S GUIDE TO PSYCHEDELIC THERAPY

LEIA FRIEDWOMAN, MS

MEDICALLY REVIEWED BY DR. DAVID COX, PHD, ABPP

Psychedelic therapy is a powerful modality that can accelerate, enhance, and deepen the therapeutic process.

By altering consciousness, psychedelic substances can help to break down barriers, foster insight, and facilitate healing. Psychedelic therapy is often used to treat conditions like addiction, PTSD, depression, and anxiety. While there are many psychedelic substances with healing potential, the ones most commonly used in therapy are psilocybin, MDMA, LSD, and ketamine. When used in the context of therapy, psychedelics have the potential to create lasting change.

Beyond this, some psychedelic medicines are not typically used in traditional therapeutic settings but show clinical efficacy for a myriad of conditions. Among these are Ayahuasca, San Pedro, N,N-Dimethyltryptamine (DMT), 5-methoxy-N,N-dimethyltryptamine (5-MeO-DMT), and ibogaine. In a legal setting, it is less common to see these psychedelics being used as agents during psychotherapy. However, people may choose to do them on their own, in a group ceremony, or at a specialized clinic (in the case of ibogaine), and then process the experience with their therapist. In such cases, individuals do not ingest the psychedelic with their therapist present, but they process the experience afterward with their therapist.

Clinical trials have investigated the applicability and efficacy of psychedelic medicine for depression, anxiety, obsessive-compulsive disorder, addiction, PTSD, and easing anxiety for patients with a terminal illness (Grob et al., 2011; Krediet et al., 2020; Moreno, Wiegand, Taitano, & Delgado, 2006; Muttoni, Ardissino, & John, 2019; Roseman, Nutt, & Carhart-Harris, 2018; Tófoli & de Araujo, 2016). Both MDMA and Psilocybin-assisted psychotherapy have been granted FDA breakthrough therapy status, a designation that expedites the process toward legalization and allows the FDA to assist researchers in the development of a promising treatment for a serious condition (M. C. Mithoefer et al., 2019; Nichols, 2020; Reiff et al., 2020). The results are limited, and some researchers say that they are cautiously optimistic (Carhart-Harris et al., 2018).

THE HISTORY OF PSYCHEDELIC THERAPY

Psychedelics were introduced to mainstream science in the 1940s and 1950s. After researchers studied them and, in some cases, self-experimented, it was determined that psychedelics were physically safe and able to be introduced into therapeutic contexts (dos Santos, Bouso, Alcázar-Córcoles, & Hallak, 2018). Humphrey Osmond, the British psychiatrist who coined the term "psychedelic" in the 1950s, found tremendous improvement in patients with alcoholism after a single LSD session, as an example.

Grinspoon and Balakar have noted that the scientists studying psychedelics were not considered counter-cultural or radical in their beliefs (Grinspoon & Bakalar, 1979). Before the Controlled Substances Act (CSA) rendered psychedelics such as LSD illegal in 1971, over 40,000 patients experienced psychedelic therapy sessions that were documented in over a thousand clinical papers.

These studies include the Spring Grove Experiment on alcoholism and LSD, the studies on mind control conducted by the CIA, the 1960 Harvard Psilocybin Project, the Concord Prison Experiment, Salvador Roquet's work with ketamine and mental health, and Dr. Stanislav Grof's early research on the heuristic and therapeutic potential of LSD and other psychedelic studies at John Hopkins University to just name a few (Bonson, 2018; Doblin, 1998; Dyck, 2005; Richard Yensen, 1996; R. Yensen, 2016). Many books were published, and six international conferences were held on psychedelic therapy. Despite evidence of their efficacy, Nixon issued the CSA, which defined LSD, psilocybin, and other psychedelics as having "significant potential for abuse and dependence" and "no recognized medicinal value." After the fact, it became known that this was a politically motivated move.

MDMA was first synthesized in 1912 by the pharmaceutical company Merck, and then in 1965 it was resynthesized by Alexander Shulgin, a chemist who created over 60 novel psychotropic compounds. Some of Shulgin's creations were excellent adjuncts to psychotherapy. MDMA was first used to assist in couples therapy.

Although psychedelic research came to a standstill after prohibition, some psychedelic therapists went underground to continue their work. However, it wasn't until 2006 that psilocybin could legally be studied in a therapeutic setting (R. R. Griffiths, Richards, McCann, & Jesse, 2006). The researchers found that when administered under supportive conditions, psilocybin could bring about mystical experiences with deep personal meaning and spiritual significance for the participants.

In 2011, the first clinical trial evaluating MDMA as an adjunct to psychotherapy found that 10 out of 12 participants had a significant reduction in PTSD symptoms (Michael C. Mithoefer, Wagner, Mithoefer, Jerome, & Doblin, 2010). This study was conducted through the Multidisciplinary Association of Psychedelic Studies, commonly referred to as MAPS. Thousands of studies investigating the effects of psilocybin and other psychedelic substances were soon to follow.

PSYCHEDELIC THERAPY'S UNIQUE PROCESS

Psychedelic therapy is a relatively new field, and as such, there is no standardized method for conducting it. Usually, some preparatory sessions take place before the actual psychedelic-assisted psychotherapy. This gives the therapist and client a chance to get to know each other and form a rapport. During these sessions, the therapist will typically explain the process of psychedelic therapy and what the client can expect. They will also discuss any concerns or questions the client may have. Once the actual therapy session begins, the therapist will usually provide guidance and assistance while the client experiences the effects of the psychedelic drug. Afterward, the therapist will help the client process and understand their experience.

There are multiple models for psychedelic therapy. A common protocol for psilocybin-assisted psychotherapy, MDMA-assisted psychotherapy, and LSD-assisted psychotherapy is non-directive with the supportive presence of a therapist or co-therapist team in a calm setting. This means that rather than being guided by a practitioner, the person is directed by the medicine and their own inner experience. Participants typically wear eyeshades, listen to evocative music, and settle into experiencing their journey. The therapist(s) remain available to talk throughout the session as needed or desired. In the days after the session, the person will typically meet with their therapist(s) and talk about what happened as well as what is coming up for them now, a process known as psychedelic integration.

On the day of the medicine session, clients typically arrive at the treatment setting in the morning. After getting situated, the client will take the medicine and lie down with eyeshades and headphones. If working with a co-therapist team, therapists may sit with one person on either side of the client, who may be lying on a bed or a couch. If working with one therapist or practitioner, that person will probably sit near the client.

Within 20-60 minutes, the psychedelic should start to take effect; this is commonly known as the "come up." The come-up lasts for under an hour; it can be a tense time, as the person's state is changing at what can feel like a rapid rate. After the come-up is the peak, the period when the client will experience the strongest subjective effects of the medicine.

The peak can last from anywhere between 1-4 hours, depending on the substance and if redosing is part of the protocol. During this time, the client may experience a range of emotions, such as fear, sadness, agitation, happiness, excitement, confusion, and more. Bodily sensations may arise, such as tingling, shaking, pressure, lightness or heaviness, temperature changes, a floaty feeling, and beyond.

During the session, the person may experience memories or visions arising in their conscious awareness. They may want to talk to their co-therapist team about what they are seeing, feeling, or thinking. In the non-directive model, therapists do not guide the client except by asking questions that may guide them toward their own inner wisdom. The therapist(s) remain as a supportive, attentive presence. According to the MAPS protocol for MDMA-assisted psychotherapy for PTSD, "An advantage of the relatively non-directive approach is that it allows each participant's process to take whichever of these paths, or any other path, chosen by the individual's innate healing intelligence" (Michael C. Mithoefer, 2017).

The therapist (s) prepare the client ahead of time about how to navigate supportive touch in sessions. If the client has expressed comfort with physical touch and consented to it ahead of time, the therapist may ask the client, "would you like me to hold your hand?"

in situations where physical contact could be supportive. Especially for psychological material related to early childhood attachment wounds and trauma, the touch may help the client to stay present to the difficult experience unfolding. Touch can be triggering, especially for clients with a history of physical or sexual trauma. Practitioners should work within their scope and participate in supervision in order to responsibly and safely provide touch in psychedelic sessions.

After the peak, the person will begin to "come down." Depending on the psychedelic, this period can last 2-5 hours or more. As the body metabolizes the psychedelic, the subjective effects become less intense. This may be a time of emotional catharsis, reflection, and processing of the experience internally or outwardly with the co-therapist team.

Ketamine-assisted psychotherapy can be done this way as well; however, a number of ketamine clinics do not provide therapy as it is not legally required that they do so, and they do not have the expertise. In clinics such as these, patients come in, receive their ketamine infusion, and go home when they feel ready. Some practitioners will prescribe ketamine lozenges so that their clients can have experiences at home. They may work with an integration therapist or provider to process what came up in the ketamine experience afterward.

Psychedelic somatic interactional psychotherapy (PSIP) is a directive therapeutic protocol that utilizes low doses of cannabis or, in rare cases, low doses of ketamine to help the person process past trauma. The person engages in an active process with their therapist throughout the session as they track sensations and emotions in the body. PSIP can also be done without any substances at all. The therapist helps the person to identify and process emotions and sensations in the body that are associated with past trauma. This modality allows the autonomic nervous system to process past trauma in a unique way.

SUBSTANCES USED IN PSYCHEDELIC THERAPY

Psychedelic therapy can be beneficial for many different conditions. There is some crossover in which psychedelic is best for what condition, and with the limited clinical research available, there are no definite answers as to what a person should take. Decades of survey research and anecdotal evidence indicate that the psychedelic experience, regardless of what catalyzes it, can have profound and long-lasting effects on a person. However, some substances may not be indicated for certain conditions.

For example, ketamine has been found to have some addictive properties when used recreationally; people have reported having trouble reducing or stopping ketamine use. This may make psychedelics such as psilocybin a better option for some people. Another example, an intense psychedelic experience without direct support during a treatment such as ayahuasca, could be retraumatizing for a person with PTSD. Clinical trials have investigated specific substances for specific conditions (such as MDMA for PTSD and psilocybin for anxiety and depression in people with terminal diagnoses) and found positive results.

Hallucinogenic drugs could trigger or worsen a pre-existing condition like bipolar disorder. If you are already diagnosed with any type of mental illness, be cautious before taking any type of psychedelic. Many professionals say that they do not recommend psychedelics for people with a personal or family history of psychosis or bipolar disorder. However, alternate perspectives (including from individuals who have been diagnosed with these conditions in the past and who use psychedelics) were presented at the Psychedelics, Madness and Awakening conference, and these bear listening to (http://www.psychedelicsmadnessawakening.com/)

Here is a list of the different types of psychedelic-assisted psychotherapy that have been investigated and some of the conditions that they may treat:

Psilocybin

- Depression and anxiety in patients with life-threatening cancer (Roland R. Griffiths et al., 2016)
- Substance use disorder (de Veen, Schellekens, Verheij, & Homberg, 2017)
- Depression and anxiety (Goldberg, Pace, Nicholas, Raison, & Hutson, 2020)
- Treatment-resistant depression (Johnson & Griffiths, 2017)
- Alcohol use disorder (Bogenschutz et al., 2018)
- Increased nature-relatedness, which could have a beneficial impact on mental health (Lyons & Carhart-Harris, 2018)
- Survey research on cluster headaches*(Schindler et al., 2015)

*Psilocybin, especially at higher doses, caused a transient headache in some healthy participants in a study (Johnson, Andrew Sewell, & Griffiths, 2012)

MDMA

- Treatment-resistant PTSD (M. C. Mithoefer et al., 2019)
- Reduction in social anxiety in autistic adults (Danforth et al., 2018)
- Couples therapy where one partner has PTSD (Almond & Allan, 2019)
- Eating disorders comorbid with PTSD (Brewerton, Lafrance, & Mithoefer, 2021)

Lysergic acid diethylamide (LSD)

- Anxiety in patients with a terminal illness (Gasser, Kirchner, & Passie, 2014)
- Alcohol use disorder (Krebs & Johansen, 2012)
- Survey research on cluster headaches (Sewell, Halpern, & Pope, 2006)

Ketamine

- Major depressive disorder (Lapidus et al., 2014)
- Substance use disorder* (Jones, Mateus, Malcolm, Brady, & Back, 2018)
- Chronic pain (Hocking & Cousins, 2003)
- Bipolar disorder (Hocking & Cousins, 2003)
- OCD (Bloch et al., 2012)
- Case studies of cluster headaches (Moisset, Clavelou, Lauxerois, Dallel, & Picard, 2017)

Ketamine use outside of a clinical setting can become addictive for some people

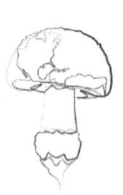

REFERENCES:

- Almond, K., & Allan, R. (2019). Incorporating MDMA as an Adjunct in Emotionally Focused Couples Therapy With Clients Impacted by Trauma or PTSD. *The Family Journal, 27*(3), 293-299. doi:10.1177/1066480719852360

- Bloch, M. H., Wasylink, S., Landeros-Weisenberger, A., Panza, K. E., Billingslea, E., Leckman, J. F., . . . Pittenger, C. (2012). Effects of Ketamine in Treatment-Refractory Obsessive-Compulsive Disorder. *Biological Psychiatry, 72*(11), 964-970. doi:https://doi.org/10.1016/j.biopsych.2012.05.028
- Bogenschutz, M. P., Podrebarac, S. K., Duane, J. H., Amegadzie, S. S., Malone, T. C., Owens, L. T., . . . Mennenga, S. E. (2018). Clinical Interpretations of Patient Experience in a Trial of Psilocybin-Assisted Psychotherapy for Alcohol Use Disorder. *Frontiers in pharmacology, 9*. doi:10.3389/fphar.2018.00100
- Bonson, K. R. (2018). Regulation of human research with LSD in the United States (1949-1987). *Psychopharmacology (Berl), 235*(2), 591-604. doi:10.1007/s00213-017-4777-4
- Brewerton, T. D., Lafrance, A., & Mithoefer, M. C. (2021). The potential use of N-methyl-3,4-methylenedioxyamphetamine (MDMA) assisted psychotherapy in the treatment of eating disorders comorbid with PTSD. *Med Hypotheses, 146*, 110367. doi:10.1016/j.mehy.2020.110367
- Carhart-Harris, R. L., Bolstridge, M., Day, C. M. J., Rucker, J., Watts, R., Erritzoe, D. E., . . . Nutt, D. J. (2018). Psilocybin with psychological support for treatment-resistant depression: six-month follow-up. *Psychopharmacology, 235*(2), 399-408. doi:10.1007/s00213-017-4771-x
- Danforth, A. L., Grob, C. S., Struble, C., Feduccia, A. A., Walker, N., Jerome, L., . . . Emerson, A. (2018). Reduction in social anxiety after MDMA-assisted psychotherapy with autistic adults: a randomized, double-blind, placebo-controlled pilot study. *Psychopharmacology, 235*(11), 3137-3148. doi:10.1007/s00213-018-5010-9

- de Veen, B. T. H., Schellekens, A. F. A., Verheij, M. M. M., & Homberg, J. R. (2017). Psilocybin for treating substance use disorders? *Expert Review of Neurotherapeutics, 17*(2), 203-212. doi:10.1080/14737175.2016.1220834
- Doblin, R. (1998). Dr. Leary's Concord Prison Experiment: a 34-year follow-up study. *J Psychoactive Drugs, 30*(4), 419-426. doi:10.1080/02791072.1998.10399715
- dos Santos, R. G., Bouso, J. C., Alcázar-Córcoles, M. Á., & Hallak, J. E. C. (2018). Efficacy, tolerability, and safety of serotonergic psychedelics for the management of mood, anxiety, and substance-use disorders: a systematic review of systematic reviews. *Expert Review of Clinical Pharmacology, 11*(9), 889-902. doi:10.1080/17512433.2018.1511424
- Dyck, E. (2005). Flashback: psychiatric experimentation with LSD in historical perspective. *Can J Psychiatry, 50*(7), 381-388. doi:10.1177/070674370505000703
- Gasser, P., Kirchner, K., & Passie, T. (2014). LSD-assisted psychotherapy for anxiety associated with a life-threatening disease: A qualitative study of acute and sustained subjective effects. *Journal of Psychopharmacology, 29*(1), 57-68. doi:10.1177/0269881114555249
- Goldberg, S. B., Pace, B. T., Nicholas, C. R., Raison, C. L., & Hutson, P. R. (2020). The experimental effects of psilocybin on symptoms of anxiety and depression: A meta-analysis. *Psychiatry research, 284*, 112749. doi:https://doi.org/10.1016/j.psychres.2020.112749
- Griffiths, R. R., Johnson, M. W., Carducci, M. A., Umbricht, A., Richards, W. A., Richards, B. D., . . . Klinedinst, M. A. (2016). Psilocybin produces substantial and sustained decreases in depression and anxiety in patients with life-threatening cancer: A randomized double-blind trial. *Journal of Psychopharmacology, 30*(12), 1181-1197. doi:10.1177/0269881116675513

- Griffiths, R. R., Richards, W. A., McCann, U., & Jesse, R. (2006). Psilocybin can occasion mystical-type experiences having substantial and sustained personal meaning and spiritual significance. *Psychopharmacology, 187*(3), 268-283. doi:10.1007/s00213-006-0457-5
- Grinspoon, L., & Bakalar, J. B. (1979). *Psychedelic drugs reconsidered* (Vol. 168): Basic Books New York.
- Grob, C. S., Danforth, A. L., Chopra, G. S., Hagerty, M., McKay, C. R., Halberstadt, A. L., & Greer, G. R. (2011). Pilot Study of Psilocybin Treatment for Anxiety in Patients With Advanced-Stage Cancer. *Archives of General Psychiatry, 68*(1), 71-78. doi:10.1001/archgenpsychiatry.2010.116
- Hocking, G., & Cousins, M. J. (2003). Ketamine in Chronic Pain Management: An Evidence-Based Review. *Anesthesia & Analgesia, 97*(6). Retrieved from https://journals.lww.com/anesthesia-analgesia/Fulltext/2003/12000/Ketamine_in_Chronic_Pain_Management__An.37.aspx
- Johnson, M. W., Andrew Sewell, R., & Griffiths, R. R. (2012). Psilocybin dose-dependently causes delayed, transient headaches in healthy volunteers. *Drug and Alcohol Dependence, 123*(1), 132-140. doi:https://doi.org/10.1016/j.drugalcdep.2011.10.029
- Johnson, M. W., & Griffiths, R. R. (2017). Potential Therapeutic Effects of Psilocybin. *Neurotherapeutics : the journal of the American Society for Experimental NeuroTherapeutics, 14*(3), 734-740. doi:10.1007/s13311-017-0542-y
- Jones, J. L., Mateus, C. F., Malcolm, R. J., Brady, K. T., & Back, S. E. (2018). Efficacy of Ketamine in the Treatment of Substance Use Disorders: A Systematic Review. *Front Psychiatry, 9*, 277. doi:10.3389/fpsyt.2018.00277

- Krebs, T. S., & Johansen, P. (2012). Lysergic acid diethylamide (LSD) for alcoholism: meta-analysis of randomized controlled trials. *Journal of psychopharmacology (Oxford, England), 26*(7), 994-1002. doi:10.1177/0269881112439253
- Krediet, E., Bostoen, T., Breeksema, J., van Schagen, A., Passie, T., & Vermetten, E. (2020). Reviewing the Potential of Psychedelics for the Treatment of PTSD. *International Journal of Neuropsychopharmacology, 23*(6), 385-400. doi:10.1093/ijnp/pyaa018
- Lapidus, K. A. B., Levitch, C. F., Perez, A. M., Brallier, J. W., Parides, M. K., Soleimani, L., . . . Murrough, J. W. (2014). A Randomized Controlled Trial of Intranasal Ketamine in Major Depressive Disorder. *Biological Psychiatry, 76*(12), 970-976. doi:https://doi.org/10.1016/j.biopsych.2014.03.026
- Lyons, T., & Carhart-Harris, R. L. (2018). Increased nature relatedness and decreased authoritarian political views after psilocybin for treatment-resistant depression. *Journal of Psychopharmacology, 32*(7), 811-819. doi:10.1177/0269881117748902
- Michael C. Mithoefer, M. D. (2017). A Manual for MDMA-Assisted Psychotherapy in the Treatment of Posttraumatic Stress Disorder, Version 8.1: . *Multidisciplinary Association for Psychedelic Studies (MAPS)*.
- Mithoefer, M. C., Feduccia, A. A., Jerome, L., Mithoefer, A., Wagner, M., Walsh, Z., . . . Doblin, R. (2019). MDMA-assisted psychotherapy for treatment of PTSD: study design and rationale for phase 3 trials based on pooled analysis of six phase 2 randomized controlled trials. *Psychopharmacology (Berl), 236*(9), 2735-2745. doi:10.1007/s00213-019-05249-5
- Mithoefer, M. C., Wagner, M. T., Mithoefer, A. T., Jerome, L., & Doblin, R. (2010). The safety and efficacy of ±3,4-methylenedioxymethamphetamine-assisted psychotherapy

in subjects with chronic, treatment-resistant posttraumatic stress disorder: the first randomized controlled pilot study. *Journal of Psychopharmacology, 25*(4), 439-452. doi:10.1177/0269881110378371
- Moisset, X., Clavelou, P., Lauxerois, M., Dallel, R., & Picard, P. (2017). Ketamine Infusion Combined With Magnesium as a Therapy for Intractable Chronic Cluster Headache: Report of Two Cases. *Headache: The Journal of Head and Face Pain, 57*(8), 1261-1264. doi:https://doi.org/10.1111/head.13135
- Moreno, F. A., Wiegand, C. B., Taitano, E. K., & Delgado, P. L. (2006). Safety, tolerability, and efficacy of psilocybin in 9 patients with obsessive-compulsive disorder. *J Clin Psychiatry, 67*(11), 1735-1740. doi:10.4088/jcp.v67n1110
- Muttoni, S., Ardissino, M., & John, C. (2019). Classical psychedelics for the treatment of depression and anxiety: A systematic review. *Journal of Affective Disorders, 258*, 11-24. doi:https://doi.org/10.1016/j.jad.2019.07.076
- Nichols, D. E. (2020). Psilocybin: from ancient magic to modern medicine. *J Antibiot (Tokyo), 73*(10), 679-686. doi:10.1038/s41429-020-0311-8
- Reiff, C. M., Richman, E. E., Nemeroff, C. B., Carpenter, L. L., Widge, A. S., Rodriguez, C. I., . . . McDonald, W. M. (2020). Psychedelics and Psychedelic-Assisted Psychotherapy. *Am J Psychiatry, 177*(5), 391-410. doi:10.1176/appi.ajp.2019.19010035
- Roseman, L., Nutt, D. J., & Carhart-Harris, R. L. (2018). Quality of Acute Psychedelic Experience Predicts Therapeutic Efficacy of Psilocybin for Treatment-Resistant Depression. *Frontiers in pharmacology, 8*. doi:10.3389/fphar.2017.00974
- Schindler, E. A. D., Gottschalk, C. H., Weil, M. J., Shapiro, R. E., Wright, D. A., & Sewell, R. A. (2015). Indoleamine Hallucinogens in Cluster Headache: Results of the

Clusterbusters Medication Use Survey. *Journal of Psychoactive Drugs, 47*(5), 372-381. doi:10.1080/02791072.2015.1107664
- Sewell, R. A., Halpern, J. H., & Pope, H. G. (2006). Response of cluster headache to psilocybin and LSD. *Neurology, 66*(12), 1920. doi:10.1212/01.wnl.0000219761.05466.43
- Tófoli, L. F., & de Araujo, D. B. (2016). Chapter Seven - Treating Addiction: Perspectives from EEG and Imaging Studies on Psychedelics. In N. M. Zahr & E. T. Peterson (Eds.), *International Review of Neurobiology* (Vol. 129, pp. 157-185): Academic Press.
- Yensen, R. (1996). The Consciousness Research of Stanislav Grof: A Cosmic Portal Beyond Individuality. In (pp. 75-84).
- Yensen, R. (2016). Psychedelic experiential psychology: pioneering clinical explorations with Salvador Roquet in The Ketamine Papers. *Multidisciplinary Association for Psychedelic Studies*, 69-93.

EIGHT
A BEGINNER'S GUIDE TO PSYCHEDELIC INTEGRATION
LEIA FRIEDWOMAN, MS

MEDICALLY REVIEWED BY DR. DAVID COX, PHD, ABPP

Psychedelic integration is the process of integrating the insights and lessons learned from a psychedelic experience into one's everyday life. For some people, this may simply mean reflecting on the experience and trying to apply its lessons. For others, it may involve more specific practices, such as journaling or meditation. Integration can be a challenge, especially if the experience was intense. However, many people find that the rewards of integration are well worth the effort. It can also bring about a deeper understanding of the interconnectedness of all things.

Integrating a journey is an important aspect of psychedelic work, and it can mean the difference between a transformational life experience and some obscure memory of a really weird night. Whether a trip happened alone, with friends, in a ceremony, in a western clinical setting, or in an indigenous shamanic one, processing these experiences is valuable.

WHAT DOES THE TERM "PSYCHEDELIC INTEGRATION" MEAN?

Psychedelic integration is a process of weaving the thread of a psychedelic experience into the tapestry of one's life, explains Dr. Katherine MacLean. On its own, a single thread can't go very far. When that thread is taken and woven together with all of the other threads that make up who we are, it becomes integrated, whole, solid, colorful work of art.

In Latin, the verb *integrare* means to form or blend into a whole or to complete. Psychedelic integration is a chance to distill the wisdom of an experience in an altered state and bring it fully into our waking lives. This allows us to keep working with the messages, giving them space to continue unfolding over time and space. Integration of the psychedelic journey may also serve to help us become more whole with ourselves.

Psychedelics have the ability to bring up repressed memories, thoughts, and emotions. For some people, this can be a difficult experience. However, it is often helpful to process this material after the fact in order to "make sense" of it. Integration can be done in a number of ways, including in a group setting, with the help of a professional therapist or coach, or on one's own. No matter what method you choose, integration can be an important step in understanding and accepting the material that was brought up during your trip.

HOW IT WORKS: INTEGRATION THERAPY, COACHING, AND CIRCLES

There is no one right way to integrate a psychedelic trip. The process can be different from person to person and can even vary from journey to journey. In the words of Julie Megler,

> "The best analogy I have for what integration really is,
> is alchemy. Each person has a unique reaction, the fires
> inside our cauldrons look different. What precipitates our

elemental reaction is an intricate and delicate process. Sometimes it leads to explosions, sometimes it leads to lead, and when we add just the right pieces, we have transformation. We can't predict what will lead to that transformation until we are in our individual cauldrons and find the pieces that melt together as a catalyst."

While the journey simmers in your cauldron, you may be thinking about how to approach your integration. Some people have the best results from integrating in a group setting. Others prefer the one-on-one attention and support of a trained professional; this option may be more appropriate for people with diagnosable conditions such as PTSD, OCD, depression, anxiety, and more. Most importantly, you should try to find the arrangement that will best alchemize your transformation.

PSYCHEDELIC INTEGRATION THERAPY

Some integration specialists are therapists, and some are coaches. The main difference between them is what responsibilities, training, and scope of practice each one has.

Psychedelic integration therapy involves working with a trained therapist to unpack prior psychedelic experience(s) and bring the wisdom of the experience into one's present reality. Therapists can work with people for the short term or on an ongoing basis. They may utilize a variety of therapeutic techniques from the domain of somatic therapy, transpersonal psychology, internal family systems, and even modalities like eye movement desensitization and reprocessing (EMDR) to help clients fully absorb and integrate the content from the psychedelic experience. With the support of the therapeutic relationship, the client can incorporate new thought, behavioral, and nervous system patterns.

Therapists undergo several years of training and practice before they receive licensure. Since the material that arises in a psychedelic trip can be incredibly personal, complex, and often related to past trauma, doing integration work with a licensed therapist can facilitate the healing process. Licensed therapists may even be able to accept your insurance for therapy, which can help keep the cost lower.

PSYCHEDELIC INTEGRATION COACHING

Psychotherapy tends to focus on looking back to see how past experiences have impacted current behaviors. Coaching differs by meeting clients where they are and focusing on the future. Coaching is a rising and unregulated field. A coach helps people reach specific, measurable goals with the intention of processing and even embracing what happened on a trip and integrating any lessons or takeaways into one's daily life.

The techniques employed by a coach or a therapist in the service of integration can look very similar; however, there are some differences between the two. Coaches cannot diagnose or treat mental disorders. They can help connect their client to information, resources, accountability, support, an objective person to help with the process, and more.

Coaches work out more tangible, specific plans with their clients, whereas the integration work with a therapist may be more open-ended and explorative of the psychological side of things. Therapists also use a diagnostic process to confirm a diagnosis and provide appropriate treatment intervention. Coaching models trade clinical intervention for client intuition and focus more on the client as an expert of themselves. Coaching models also remove a "hierarchy" of the expert-patient dynamic and come together as equals. Many coaches use a humanistic lens and may share personal details about their life and story. Therapy models typically frown upon self-disclosure, which can also impact the client-therapist relationship.

While therapists are held accountable by a licensure board, continuing education, and a code of ethics, anyone can call themselves a coach. This lower barrier to entry can be beneficial, as not everyone has the means or access to complete all the schooling necessary to become a therapist. Indeed, someone can be an amazing support to people without going through 7+ years of school. However, it also creates a dangerous circumstance where untrained individuals help clients hold their deep traumas and pains. Many coaches go through trauma-informed programs to teach them how to work effectively and ethically with people.

Consider asking a prospective coach if they are engaged in a community of practice with peer supervision and mentorship from seasoned practitioners.

If you have trauma (we all do, to varying degrees), ask if the prospective practitioner is trauma-informed, meaning they have special training and certifications in emotional trauma, trauma and the central nervous system, dissociation, panic, somatic work, and/or PTSD.

INTEGRATION CIRCLES

Integration circles provide a supportive container for people to share insights and experiences from altered consciousness states in a group setting. Listening to others' stories and hearing how they are working through their own processes can be just as valuable as sharing one's own story. In a circle, the collective wisdom of the group can emerge through the sharing of stories, experiences, emotions, and feelings. These circles can offer a space for emotional processing, catharsis, and deep connection with others.

The experience of being witnessed and heard by others in a non-judgmental and supportive way can be healing and transformative.

There are many integration circles one can find online to attend. Some are facilitated by therapists, coaches, or peers. Some circles are non-hierarchical, and the duties of facilitation shift from person to person.

PRACTICAL STRATEGIES FOR INTEGRATING A PSYCHEDELIC EXPERIENCE

After a trip, there may be physical, emotional, mental, or even spiritual material to process. Integration is unique to each person and trip; perhaps it starts with going over notes or voice recordings from the journey and talking about it with the sitter, therapist(s), or friend who was there. Spending time alone, spending time in nature, journaling current thoughts and feelings, creating art or writing that expresses an aspect of the journey, such as visions or felt sensations, and moving the body are great places to start.

It may be illuminating to pay attention to one's thoughts, feelings, and urges in the days following a trip. One can try to observe and accept what is present there rather than try to change it or react to it.

Dreams may be especially strange and potent after a psychedelic trip, so some people write down their dreams and look at what messages might be bubbling up from the unconscious mind.

Integration is a great time to examine behaviors with a compassionately critical eye and decide what to let go of, as well as any behaviors to cultivate and hone.

In the Psychedelic Medicine Integration Workbook, Kaufman and McCamy emphasize that integration is a journey, not a destination (Kaufman & McCamy, 2020). They put forth the Ayavolve Integration

Model for the process of psychedelic healing work, which includes a five-step process:

Work with plant medicine/psychedelic → Insights and processing of ceremony experiences → Digest the healing and learning → Take actions → The self evolves.

In this way, the psychedelic experience is only one aspect of a journey toward evolution. A person will not necessarily access self-evolution unless they have taken the time to process the material from the journey and taken meaningful steps to apply that wisdom to their life.

The Psychedelic Medicine Integration Workbook also suggests examining the psychedelic experience through the lens of categories, including body, mind, visions, emotions, memories, and themes.

SOME QUESTIONS INCLUDE:

- What sensations did you feel inside your body?
- What emotions did you feel? (e.g.: sadness, grief, anger, fear, jealousy, joy, gratitude, frustration)
- Did any memories come up during the process?
- What were your thoughts during the experience?
- Did you notice any patterns about yourself and your behavior?
- Did you have any visions?
- Were there any interpersonal dynamics from the experience that should be explored? Are there things that came up that you would like clarification from the facilitators, group

members, sitter, or whoever was with you for the experience?
- Did anything else happen that feels worthy of noting?

After processing the experience, the next step may be to look forward and consider how this experience could be applied to your life. Questions to meditate on, adapted from the Workbook, include:

- What realization(s) or insight(s) came from the experience?
- What do you now feel you need to work on most in your life?
- Did your experience match up with the original intention that you set?
- How can you integrate the lessons that you learned into your daily life?
- What form of expression might you use to articulate the unique experience you had? Do you feel called to journaling, meditation, movement, singing, or any other form of expression?
- Consider how you can express aspects of your journey to other people. Is there anything specific that you want to share with someone, or anything that you *don't* want to share?

Psychedelics can increase nature-relatedness (Kettner, Gandy, Haijen, & Carhart-Harris, 2019). Some people find that being outside and interacting with nature supports their integration process. Research suggests that mindfulness training coupled with psychedelic integration has been effective at increasing feelings of mental health and well-being (Payne, Chambers, & Liknaitzky, 2021). It may be beneficial to learn about mindfulness and practice some techniques in support of an integration process.

A NOTE ABOUT ONE-NESS

Psychedelic experiences can catalyze states of ego-dissolution or a feeling of being "one with everything." Psychedelics can also make a person feel as though they are completely alone in the universe. Whether a person has had an experience on one or both ends of that spectrum, considering how to give back to the world can also be part of the integration.

COMPLETE YOUR EXPERIENCE WITH PSYCHEDELIC INTEGRATION PRACTICES

The experience of a psychedelic can often be overwhelming and jarring, leading to what some have termed "ego death." This can be a disorienting experience, but it also offers the opportunity for tremendous growth and transformation. During integration, individuals have the chance to reflect on their experiences and find ways to incorporate the insights they've gained into their daily lives. This process is often helped by working with a therapist or other professional, as well as by talking about the experience with trusted friends or others who have had similar experiences. Integration can be a challenging process, but it ultimately offers a unique opportunity for personal growth and enrichment.

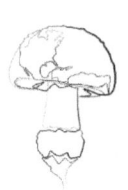

REFERENCES:

- Kaufman, D. R., & McCamy, M. (2020). The Psychedelic Medicine Integration Workbook.
- Kettner, H., Gandy, S., Haijen, E. C. H. M., & Carhart-Harris, R. L. (2019). From Egoism to Ecoism: Psychedelics Increase Nature Relatedness in a State-Mediated and Context-Dependent Manner. *International Journal of Environmental Research and Public Health, 16*(24), 5147. Retrieved from https://www.mdpi.com/1660-4601/16/24/5147
- Payne, J. E., Chambers, R., & Liknaitzky, P. (2021). Combining Psychedelic and Mindfulness Interventions: Synergies to Inform Clinical Practice. *ACS Pharmacology & Translational Science, 4*(2), 416-423. doi:10.1021/acsptsci.1c00034

NINE
A BEGINNER'S GUIDE TO MICRODOSING
AMBER KRAUS

MEDICALLY REVIEWED BY DR. DAVID COX, PHD, ABPP

Microdosing is the act of taking very small amounts of a psychedelic drug in order to achieve subtle yet noticeable effects on mood, creativity, and overall well-being. Although it is not a new phenomenon, the practice has gained popularity in recent years due largely to media attention and the emergence of online microdosing communities. Psychedelics, including LSD and psilocybin (commonly known as "magic mushrooms"), are widely used for this purpose, and there are chapters devoted to microdosing each in this book.

Despite the lack of scientific research on microdosing, some studies suggest it could improve cognitive function (Prochazkova et al., 2018). Psychedelics are thought to work by modulating neurotransmitter signaling, and it is believed that microdoses may produce subtle changes in brain function that contribute to the therapeutic effects reported by users.

WHAT IS MICRODOSING?

Microdosing involves using a sub-perceptible amount of psychedelic drugs to improve mood or enhance cognitive performance in work and play while eliminating the physiological experiences associated with "tripping" (an increase in heart rate, changes in vision, perceptions of time, etc.).

The goal of microdosing is to develop practical applications for psychedelic substances in everyday life. Its increasing popularity may be attributed partially to the fact that microdosers claim they can experience the benefits of the psychedelic substance of their choice *without* the perception-altering effects of a full dose of psychedelic. Considering that most long-term benefits of psychedelic therapy are attributed to the trip and integration of the experience, microdosing operates from a different therapeutic paradigm.

Scientific research is in the beginning stages, but much of the research on microdosing is mainly anecdotal or self-reported survey research. A recent study suggests that the benefits of microdosing can also be attributed to the placebo effect (Szigeti et al., 2021). With 191 participants, this study was the most extensive placebo-controlled study that has been done on psychedelics. The results found that while the microdose group reported improved psychological outcomes, so did the placebo group, with little difference between the two. There have been other recent cross-sectional studies that have identified improvements in mood (Anderson et al., 2019; Johnstad, 2018; Lea et al., 2020; Szigeti et al., 2021; Webb, Copes, & Hendricks, 2019), cognitive function (Lea et al., 2020; Rosenbaum et al., 2020; Webb et al., 2019), reductions in stress (Polito & Stevenson, 2019), depression (Cameron, Nazarian, & Olson, 2020; Polito & Stevenson, 2019; Webb et al., 2019), and anxiety (Cameron et al., 2020; Kaertner et al., 2021; Lea et al., 2020; Polito & Stevenson, 2019).

IS MICRODOSING RIGHT FOR ME?

One of the reasons people microdose is for its potential benefits on mental health. The science around microdosing is still being explored, but one study suggests it may help with depression, anxiety, and other psychological disorders (Polito & Stevenson, 2019). Microdosing may also improve creativity and enhance one's overall outlook on life. Although more research is needed to understand the risks and benefits of microdosing, it is a practice that continues to gain popularity. As society becomes increasingly open to alternative forms of medicine, it is likely that more people will explore microdosing as a way to improve their mental and physical health.

MICRODOSING TO INCREASE PRODUCTIVITY & CREATIVITY

One of the most popular reasons people give for microdosing is to improve focus, creativity, and productivity (Anderson et al., 2019). In today's fast-paced world, where it can seem that self-worth is increasingly dependent on productivity and outputs, young professionals are looking for ways to stand out from their peers. It has become a popular trend among Silicon Valley professionals looking to gain a competitive edge in their field.

Those who microdose regularly report that it makes them feel more productive in their work, more able to focus, and enhances their creativity. One San Francisco professional says, "It helps me think more creatively and stay focused. I manage my stress with ease and am able to keep my perspective healthy in a way that I was unable to before."

MICRODOSING FOR DEPRESSION & ANXIETY

While research demonstrates that psychedelic therapy is helpful in cases of depression and anxiety, there is no clinical evidence of the impacts of microdosing on depression and anxiety (Kuypers, 2020).

A review of low-dose psilocybin and LSD studies suggests that there is potential for smaller doses of psychedelics to serve as a treatment option for otherwise healthy individuals who are struggling with depression or anxiety. A microdose of some psychedelics could affect cognitive flexibility by reducing the tendency toward rumination, a thinking pattern commonly experienced as a symptom of depression.

The idea is that when taken at low doses, psychedelics can improve mood and productivity while reducing the risk of harmful side effects, like anxiety, that might be experienced during a full-blown trip. On the day following a trip, some people might experience feelings of depression as their neurotransmitters recalibrate. If microdosing, there may not be as much of a risk of post-trip depression.

With microdosing, it's not about altering consciousness—it's about using psychedelic drugs to improve everyday life. Novelist Alayet Waldman, who has suffered from mood disorders for most of her life, did a 30-day microdosing experiment with LSD and wrote about it in her book *A Really Good Day: How Microdosing Made a Mega Difference in My Mood, My Marriage, and My Life* (Waldman, 2018). On her first day taking a microdose of LSD, she wrote about how normal she felt. "I'm content and relaxed. I'm busy, but not stressed. That might be normal for some people, but it isn't for me." For many people who struggle with mood disorders such as anxiety and depression, this is the ultimate goal: to have a "really good day."

MICRODOSING FOR PAIN RELIEF

Research by the Beckley Foundation, an organization focused on global drug policy reform and psychedelic drug research, conducted a study to determine if low doses of psychedelic drugs such as LSD could be used as a non-addictive pain management technique. In their 2020 study, researchers provided 24 individuals with a single dose of 5, 10, or 20 micrograms of LSD or a placebo (Ramaekers et al., 2020). The study found that the 20-microgram dose consistently increased pain tolerance by 20% compared to the placebo group. However, it is worth noting that the 5 and 10-microgram doses did not have the same effects.

The study noted that the perceptive pain tolerance while under the influence of the 20-microgram dose of LSD was comparable to the effects of opioids such as oxycodone and morphine. This study also showed that the pain reduction effects of a 20-microgram dose may have extended beyond the five-hour study window. This could be a significant breakthrough in the world of pain management.

HOW MUCH IS A MICRODOSE?

One of the most critical aspects of microdosing is to ensure proper dosage. Too much, and a person runs the risk of experiencing a full psychedelic trip, which likely isn't the intended outcome before walking into a board meeting or while in the middle of a project deadline.

In clinical settings, a microdose would consist of 10–20 mcg of LSD and/or 0.3–0.5 g of psilocybin-containing mushrooms. That is roughly 1/10th of a typical active dose. For most people starting microdosing, they begin with 50-100mg for a very mild experience, 100-150mg to feel it slightly, and 200-250mg to definitely feel it. The goal is to use psychedelics in a way that reduces the risk of having an intense experience. This allows people to go about their day as if nothing was very different.

Many people choose to grind their mushrooms up and create their own capsules. By doing this, they blend the inconsistencies in psilocybin between cap and stems. Cap-M-Quick is a popular capsule filler that makes this process painless.

HOW DO I SCHEDULE MY MICRODOSES?

The most common protocol for microdosing can be attributed to James Fadiman, an American psychologist and author of *The Psychedelic Explorer's Guide*, who is well known for his work in psychedelic research (Fadiman, 2011; Fadiman & Korb, 2019). Fadiman collected thousands of anecdotal reports and has been active in promoting scientific research into the benefits of microdosing. While his protocol was originally created to microdose with LSD, it can also be used for psilocybin. He suggests starting with 1/20 to 1/10 of a recreational dose of the substance of choice and dose every three days with two rest days in between. At the end of each thirty-day cycle, rest for two weeks.

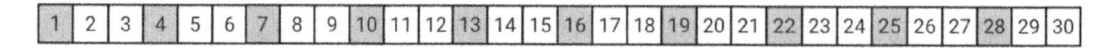

| 1 | 2 | 3 | 4 | 5 | 6 | 7 | 8 | 9 | 10 | 11 | 12 | 13 | 14 | 15 | 16 | 17 | 18 | 19 | 20 | 21 | 22 | 23 | 24 | 25 | 26 | 27 | 28 | 29 | 30 |

Fadiman Protocol: Take a microdose every 3rd day. At the end of each thirty-day cycle, rest for two weeks.

The other popular protocol for microdosing was developed by world-renowned mycologist Paul Stamets. With the Stamets protocol, people microdose for four consecutive days, followed by a three-day break. This is continued for one month, followed by a 2-4-week rest period to notice any changes and allow for a body reset.

Stamets recommends microdosing with a combination of Lion's Mane, niacin (B3), and psilocybin. His specific stack designed to repair, rebuild, and enhance creativity and cognitive function for a 154-pound person is:

- 100 mg psilocybin
- 200-500 mg lion's mane mushroom extract
- 100-200 mg niacin

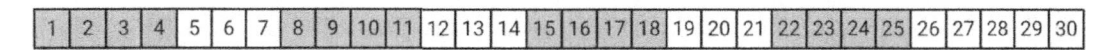

1	2	3	4	5	6	7	8	9	10	11	12	13	14	15	16	17	18	19	20	21	22	23	24	25	26	27	28	29	30

Stamets Protocol: Take a microdose every day for four days in a row and then rest for three. Take a 2-4 week break after every month.

WHAT TO DO IF YOU ACCIDENTALLY MACRODOSE

It is not uncommon to accidentally take too much psilocybin or LSD, especially when first starting to microdose. If this happens, the first recommendation is to not panic and to enjoy the journey. If you feel that you have accidentally macrodosed, you may want to remove yourself from work or other social situations and rest somewhere comfortable and safe. Many people choose to put on headphones and listen to calm, meditative music. Keep in mind everything else you have read about the safety of psychedelics in this book, and trust that this unplanned experience will end.

RISKS ASSOCIATED WITH MICRODOSING

Despite a positive outlook, microdosing is generally considered safe but does have some risks. These range from difficulty concentrating to unexpected such as increased anxiety and physiological discomfort

Those who have been diagnosed with psychotic disorders such as schizophrenia or bipolar disorder are discouraged from using psychedelic drugs at any dosage, as negative consequences may be experienced. Microdosing has been shown to increase neuroticism in one self-reported study, but these results have not been validated in clinical trials. This being said, in a recent discussion between James Fadiman and Sam Harris, Fadiman mentioned three things specifically related to this topic: First, there is little to no research on psychedelics on people with schizophrenia or bipolar disorders as they introduce a level of risk that researchers have not been willing to take; second, there are thousands of self-reported anecdotes from people with bipolar disorder who have used psychedelics. Third, those that have reported typically say it is not a good idea to use them in a manic state and that positive experiences have been had while in a depressive state.

It is always a good idea to do thorough research before mixing any drugs, including prescription drugs that are taken regularly. If you are currently taking antidepressant medications, it is highly recommended that you get guidance from a psychiatrist prior to microdosing. Microdosing is also not advisable for people who are colorblind, have chronic anxiety, or are on the autism spectrum.

When considering psychedelic drug use in any form, the substance should always be tested for purity. When using any psychedelic substance outside of a clinical setting, it is possible that the substance could be cut with other potentially lethal contaminants. There are harm-reduction networks where testing kits can be accessed that will indicate whether a substance is pure or not.

MICRODOSING IS ILLEGAL IN THE UNITED STATES

A significant risk with microdosing is that most psychedelic drugs are illegal to use outside of clinical settings in the United States and many other countries. This means that it can be difficult or impossible to obtain psychedelics for microdosing purposes from a legal source. As a result, it is important to be aware of the source of any psychedelic substances that are used for microdosing.

MICRODOSING: A SCIENTIFIC MEANS FOR ENHANCING WELL-BEING, OR A TRENDY PLACEBO EFFECT?

Although it is not yet been backed by scientific research, anecdotal reports suggest that microdosing has a host of potential benefits, including increased creativity, focus, and energy levels. For those looking to microdose, it is important to measure substances precisely to avoid accidentally *macrodosing*—that is, taking enough of the substance to experience a change in conscious perception. It is also helpful to solicit the advice of an experienced guide who can provide recommendations for a microdosing schedule. With careful consideration and planning, microdosing can be an effective way to enhance well-being.

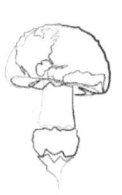

REFERENCES:

- Anderson, T., Petranker, R., Rosenbaum, D., Weissman, C. R., Dinh-Williams, L. A., Hui, K., . . . Farb, N. A. S. (2019). Microdosing psychedelics: personality, mental health, and creativity differences in microdosers. *Psychopharmacology (Berl), 236*(2), 731-740. doi:10.1007/s00213-018-5106-2
- Cameron, L. P., Nazarian, A., & Olson, D. E. (2020). Psychedelic Microdosing: Prevalence and Subjective Effects. *J Psychoactive Drugs, 52*(2), 113-122. doi:10.1080/02791072.2020.1718250
- Fadiman, J. (2011). *The psychedelic explorer's guide: Safe, therapeutic, and sacred journeys*: Simon and Schuster.
- Fadiman, J., & Korb, S. (2019). Might Microdosing Psychedelics Be Safe and Beneficial? An Initial Exploration. *Journal of Psychoactive Drugs, 51*(2), 118-122. doi:10.1080/02791072.2019.1593561
- Johnstad, P. G. (2018). Powerful substances in tiny amounts: an interview study of psychedelic microdosing. *Nordic Studies on Alcohol and Drugs, 35*(1), 39-51.
- Kaertner, L. S., Steinborn, M. B., Kettner, H., Spriggs, M. J., Roseman, L., Buchborn, T., . . . Carhart-Harris, R. L. (2021). Positive expectations predict improved mental-health outcomes linked to psychedelic microdosing. *Scientific Reports, 11*(1), 1941. doi:10.1038/s41598-021-81446-7
- Kuypers, K. P. C. (2020). The therapeutic potential of microdosing psychedelics in depression. *Ther Adv Psychopharmacol, 10*, 2045125320950567. doi:10.1177/2045125320950567
- Lea, T., Amada, N., Jungaberle, H., Schecke, H., Scherbaum, N., & Klein, M. (2020). Perceived outcomes of psychedelic microdosing as self-managed therapies for mental and substance use disorders. *Psychopharmacology, 237*(5), 1521-1532. doi:10.1007/s00213-020-05477-0
- Polito, V., & Stevenson, R. J. (2019). A systematic study of microdosing psychedelics. *PloS one, 14*(2), e0211023-

- e0211023. doi:10.1371/journal.pone.0211023
- Prochazkova, L., Lippelt, D. P., Colzato, L. S., Kuchar, M., Sjoerds, Z., & Hommel, B. (2018). Exploring the effect of microdosing psychedelics on creativity in an open-label natural setting. *Psychopharmacology, 235*(12), 3401-3413. doi:10.1007/s00213-018-5049-7
- Ramaekers, J. G., Hutten, N., Mason, N. L., Dolder, P., Theunissen, E. L., Holze, F., . . . Kuypers, K. P. C. (2020). A low dose of lysergic acid diethylamide decreases pain perception in healthy volunteers. *Journal of Psychopharmacology, 35*(4), 398-405. doi:10.1177/0269881120940937
- Rootman, J. M., Kiraga, M., Kryskow, P., Harvey, K., Stamets, P., Santos-Brault, E., . . . Walsh, Z. (2022). Psilocybin microdosers demonstrate greater observed improvements in mood and mental health at one month relative to non-microdosing controls. *Scientific Reports, 12*(1), 11091. doi:10.1038/s41598-022-14512-3
- Rootman, J. M., Kryskow, P., Harvey, K., Stamets, P., Santos-Brault, E., Kuypers, K. P. C., . . . Walsh, Z. (2021). Adults who microdose psychedelics report health related motivations and lower levels of anxiety and depression compared to non-microdosers. *Sci Rep, 11*(1), 22479. doi:10.1038/s41598-021-01811-4
- Rosenbaum, D., Weissman, C., Anderson, T., Petranker, R., Dinh-Williams, L.-A., Hui, K., & Hapke, E. (2020). Microdosing psychedelics: demographics, practices, and psychiatric comorbidities. *Journal of Psychopharmacology, 34*(6), 612-622.
- Szigeti, B., Kartner, L., Blemings, A., Rosas, F., Feilding, A., Nutt, D. J., . . . Erritzoe, D. (2021). Self-blinding citizen science to explore psychedelic microdosing. *Elife, 10*. doi:10.7554/eLife.62878

- Waldman, A. (2018). *A really good day: how microdosing made a mega difference in my mood, my marriage, and my life*: Anchor.
- Webb, M., Copes, H., & Hendricks, P. S. (2019). Narrative identity, rationality, and microdosing classic psychedelics. *International Journal of Drug Policy, 70*, 33-39.

TEN
WHERE DO I START?
MATT ZEMON, MSC

MEDICALLY REVIEWED BY DR. DAVID FLYNN, MD, MBA, CPHQ

"Where do I start" is the most common question people ask who are interested in psychedelics but are unsure of where to begin. This is an incredibly personal question and, because of the many variables at play, one of the reasons why I put this book together.

At the same time, I recognize the need for a "cheat sheet" that condenses 400 pages down to four. In an effort to be helpful, I have taken some of the information that you will find as you read on and summarized them in this chapter.

Please note, I am not advising you to try anything. This chapter is a summary of two of the top choices people are making for each category and some of the reasons why.

FOR PEOPLE INTERESTED IN PSYCHEDELIC-ASSISTED THERAPY:

Please make sure you read Leia Friedwoman's chapter, "A Beginner's Guide to Psychedelic Therapy," where she walks through psychedelic therapy, the various substances, what they are being used for, and how the process works. In the meantime, here are some brief thoughts:

Option 1: Ketamine

With a prescription, ketamine is legal in the United States and is being used on and off-label to treat everything from anxiety and depression to substance use disorder to chronic pain and cluster headaches. This medicine is being used by people who do not respond to traditional antidepressants such as SSRIs, as well as those who prefer not to take a daily medication. Unlike the other psychedelic medicines, ketamine can also be taken in conjunction with SSRIs.

Cost is one of the most significant barriers to ketamine treatment. Insurers don't typically pay for it, and ketamine infusions can cost between $400 to $2,000 per treatment. Esketamine nasal spray, which can be covered by insurance, typically costs between $590 and $885 per treatment session. Companies like HAPPŸŸ, Mindbloom, and nue.life have brought the cost down to closer to $200 per treatment by prescribing via telehealth and having the patients take their treatment at home. While less expensive, more responsibility falls on the patients.

Option 2: Psilocybin and MDMA

MDMA, commonly referred to as "ecstasy" or "molly," and psilocybin, also known as "magic mushrooms," are used legally in the United States in FDA-approved clinical research studies on patients with depression, substance use disorders (including smoking), and other mental health conditions, but it is not yet available to the general public. The FDA has given both drugs "Breakthrough Therapy" designations (Mithoefer et al., 2019; Nichols, 2020; Reiff et al., 2020). MDMA is currently part of a Phase

3 study specifically for patients with severe, chronic post-traumatic stress disorder (PTSD) sponsored by the nonprofit Multidisciplinary Association for Psychedelic Studies (MAPS). Of participants who received three MDMA-assisted therapy sessions, 67% no longer qualified for a PTSD diagnosis, and 88% experienced a clinically meaningful reduction in symptoms (Feder et al., 2021).

To receive treatments with these substances, a person must qualify to participate in a specific clinical trial. People who do not qualify for a clinical trial can potentially get access through an "expanded access" program. Terminally ill patients can work with their doctors to petition the FDA for compassionate use of investigational drugs. Patients in the US with immediately life-threatening diseases or conditions can also petition drug developers for access to investigational drugs under the Right to Try Act. Terminally ill Canadian patients can now be treated with psilocybin and MDMA through their "Special Access Program" with a 56(1) exemption.

In 2020, Oregon voted to legalize the therapeutic use of psilocybin and is working to create regulations to govern how this will be implemented. MAPS is hopeful that the results of the MDMA study will result in FDA approval in 2023.

For those with the resources to travel, Psilocybin retreats are legal in the Bahamas, Brazil, Jamaica, and the Netherlands (as a truffle). In Mexico, retreats are technically illegal, but this has been unenforced when used in ceremony settings. As with all things in this book, readers are strongly suggested to research thoroughly.

FOR PEOPLE INTERESTED IN EXPANDING CONSCIOUSNESS:

Psychedelic medicine's ability to create a spiritual experience is well-documented. In a 2019 Johns Hopkins survey of 4,285 people who reported personal experiences with God either on their own or with the use of a psychedelic, more than two-thirds of self-identified Atheists dropped the Atheist label afterward (Griffiths, Hurwitz, Davis, Johnson, & Jesse, 2019).

Dr. Stanislav Grof, MD, PhD, has spent 60 years studying consciousness, has accompanied close to 4,000 individual psychedelic sessions with patients, and has written 22 books and 160 articles on the theoretical and practical implications of modern consciousness research for psychiatry, psychology, and psychotherapy. He refers to the non-ordinary states attained with psychedelics as "holotropic" (Grof, 1998). This composite word means oriented or moving toward wholeness. In his seasoned opinion, holotropic techniques, including psychedelic medicines, allow contact between the conscious ego and the spiritual consciousness. In *The Consciousness Revolution*, he writes, "…in these states it is possible to encounter a rich array of experiences which are very similar to those that inspired the great religions of the world – visions of God and various divine and demonic beings, encounters with discarnate entities, episodes of psycho-spiritual death and rebirth, visits to Heaven and Hell, past life experiences, and many others" (Grof, 2010).

Brother David Steindl-Rast is a Benedictine monk with a PhD in experimental psychology who has studied with Zen masters and dedicated most of his life to interfaith dialogue. He told the *Los Angeles Times* that his experience with psychedelics was "like climbing all day in the fog and then suddenly, briefly seeing the mountain peak for the first time. There are no shortcuts to the awakened attitude, and it takes daily work and effort. But the drug gives you a vision, a glimpse of what you are seeking."

Dr. Carlos Warter, MD, PhD, who wrote the forward to this book, has described psychedelics, when done with intention and preparation, as an "initiation into consciousness." Brian C. Muraresku, the author of the *New York Times* Bestseller, *The Immortality Key*, has spent twelve years researching and documenting the role psychedelic drugs have played in the origins of

Western civilization and, more specifically, Christianity. There are connections between psychedelics and almost every major religion, as Sophie Saint Thomas explores in her "Do the World's Biggest Religions have Psychedelic Origins" contribution.

For those interested in exploring consciousness further for themselves, I encourage you to begin by reading the entire Psychedelics 101 chapter and *How to Change Your Mind* by Michael Pollan. While all psychedelics can be used for expanding consciousness, I am lifting up two of the most common starting options.

Option 1: Ketamine

To be legal in the United States, ketamine must be used in conjunction with anxiety and/or depression treatment. While ketamine must be prescribed, there are psychologists, therapists, guides, and spiritual leaders across the world who can assist in the preparation and integration components of using ketamine for expanding consciousness. Many practitioners can be found in online directories such as those published by Psychable.com, MAPS.org, Tripsitters.org, and Psychedelics.support. There are also more than 100 psychedelic societies and groups where people meet regularly for education and support purposes. The quality of practitioners varies widely, so please do your research.

Option 2: Psilocybin or Ayahuasca Retreats

Legal (and sometimes not legal) consciousness retreats for all budgets are available in many countries worldwide, including Costa Rica, Mexico, Jamaica, the Netherlands, Ecuador, and Peru. If this interests you, I would recommend reading Leia Friedwoman's "Finding your Ayahuasca Retreat" and "Sexual abuse in psychedelic ceremonies." There are also two American churches (Uniao Do

Vegetal and Santo Daime) that are allowed to consume Ayahuasca under the Religious Freedom Restoration Act. The Oklevueha Native American Church also provides ayahuasca ceremonies in the United States, but, as indigenous people did not found it, the church has had legitimacy challenges.

Underground (illegal) retreats take place all over the United States. Before considering participating in one of these, it is highly recommended that the retreat leaders are carefully vetted for experience, training, and how they handle challenging situations.

For those considering a peyote ceremony, please consider San Pedro and read "Why Peyote Sustainability Matters" and "Peyote Legality and Religious Freedom: A Primer for Settlers," by Alice de Witt.

FOR PEOPLE INTERESTED IN PSYCHEDELICS FOR SUBSTANCE USE CHALLENGES:

Option 1: Ketamine

A significant amount of research has been published lately on the use of ketamine for substance use challenges, including Ivan Ezquerra-Romano and colleagues, "Ketamine For the Treatment of Addiction," published in *Neuropharmacology (Ivan Ezquerra-Romano, Lawn, Krupitsky, & Morgan, 2018)*, a systematic review of "Efficacy of Ketamine in the Treatment of Substance Use Disorders" by Jones et al., published in *Front Psychiatry (Jones, Mateus, Malcolm, Brady, & Back, 2018)*, and "Ketamine Psychedelic Therapy (KPT): A review of the Results of Ten Years of Research" by Krupitsky & Grinenko, published in the *Journal of Psychoactive Drugs (Krupitsky & Grinenko, 1997)*.

Option 2: Ibogaine

Ibogaine is most known for its ability to eliminate withdrawals from opiates and is showing promise for other drug withdrawal symptoms as well. People have self-reported complete elimination of withdrawal symptoms within one to two hours of ingestion from substances such as heroin. Reports also reveal a reduction in drug cravings, potentially lowering the risk of ongoing drug use among people with narcotic dependencies. In addition to opiate treatment, peer-reviewed journals are highlighting the benefits of using ibogaine to treat addiction to stimulants, including nicotine, methamphetamine, and alcohol (Brown, Noller, & Denenberg, 2019; Heink, Katsikas, & Lange-Altman, 2017; Schenberg et al., 2017).

Treatment with ibogaine carries more health risks than other psychedelics, and finding a safe, experienced ibogaine treatment center is essential (Litjens & Brunt, 2016; Noller, Frampton, & Yazar-Klosinski, 2018). The most common ways to gain access to ibogaine therapy are:

- Partake in a traditional ceremony with Bwiti providers either in Gabon or with those initiated into Bwiti, the West African belief system where iboga root bark is a rite of passage. Note: These centers usually have more experience with people seeking psycho-spiritual guidance rather than substance abuse and use Iboga rather than the extract ibogaine.
- Holistic and therapeutic medically monitored centers, where the provider usually has completed an apprenticeship at another ibogaine treatment center, fully staffed with medical personnel, therapists and counselors, apprentices, and ibogaine providers.
- Clinical treatment centers operated out of medical centers and hospitals.

While illegal in the United States, there are ibogaine treatment centers in many countries around the world.

For more information on ibogaine, please look at the ibogaine chapter and the various contributions by Shea Prueger and Katie Stone.

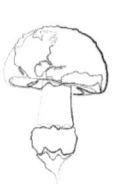

REFERENCES:

- Brown, T. K., Noller, G. E., & Denenberg, J. O. (2019). Ibogaine and Subjective Experience: Transformative States and Psychopharmacotherapy in the Treatment of Opioid Use Disorder. *J Psychoactive Drugs, 51*(2), 155-165. doi:10.1080/02791072.2019.1598603
- Feder, A., Costi, S., Rutter, S. B., Collins, A. B., Govindarajulu, U., Jha, M. K., . . . Charney, D. S. (2021). A Randomized Controlled Trial of Repeated Ketamine Administration for Chronic Posttraumatic Stress Disorder. *Am J Psychiatry, 178*(2), 193-202. doi:10.1176/appi.ajp.2020.20050596
- Griffiths, R. R., Hurwitz, E. S., Davis, A. K., Johnson, M. W., & Jesse, R. (2019). Survey of subjective "God encounter experiences": Comparisons among naturally occurring experiences and those occasioned by the classic psychedelics psilocybin, LSD, ayahuasca, or DMT. *PloS one, 14*(4), e0214377-e0214377. doi:10.1371/journal.pone.0214377

- Grof, S. (1998). Human nature and the nature of reality: conceptual challenges from consciousness research. *J Psychoactive Drugs, 30*(4), 343-357. doi:10.1080/02791072.1998.10399710
- Grof, S. (2010). *The consciousness revolution: New perspectives in psychiatry, psychology, and psychotherapy.* Paper presented at the Proceedings of the seventeenth international transpersonal conference.
- Heink, A., Katsikas, S., & Lange-Altman, T. (2017). Examination of the Phenomenology of the Ibogaine Treatment Experience: Role of Altered States of Consciousness and Psychedelic Experiences. *J Psychoactive Drugs, 49*(3), 201-208. doi:10.1080/02791072.2017.1290855
- Ivan Ezquerra-Romano, I., Lawn, W., Krupitsky, E., & Morgan, C. J. A. (2018). Ketamine for the treatment of addiction: Evidence and potential mechanisms. *Neuropharmacology, 142,* 72-82. doi:10.1016/j.neuropharm.2018.01.017
- Jones, J. L., Mateus, C. F., Malcolm, R. J., Brady, K. T., & Back, S. E. (2018). Efficacy of Ketamine in the Treatment of Substance Use Disorders: A Systematic Review. *Front Psychiatry, 9,* 277. doi:10.3389/fpsyt.2018.00277
- Krupitsky, E. M., & Grinenko, A. Y. (1997). Ketamine Psychedelic Therapy (KPT): A Review of the Results of Ten Years of Research. *Journal of Psychoactive Drugs, 29*(2), 165-183. doi:10.1080/02791072.1997.10400185
- Litjens, R. P., & Brunt, T. M. (2016). How toxic is ibogaine? *Clin Toxicol (Phila), 54*(4), 297-302. doi:10.3109/15563650.2016.1138226
- Mithoefer, M. C., Feduccia, A. A., Jerome, L., Mithoefer, A., Wagner, M., Walsh, Z., . . . Doblin, R. (2019). MDMA-assisted psychotherapy for treatment of PTSD: study design and rationale for phase 3 trials based on pooled

- analysis of six phase 2 randomized controlled trials. *Psychopharmacology (Berl), 236*(9), 2735-2745. doi:10.1007/s00213-019-05249-5
- Nichols, D. E. (2020). Psilocybin: from ancient magic to modern medicine. *J Antibiot (Tokyo), 73*(10), 679-686. doi:10.1038/s41429-020-0311-8
- Noller, G. E., Frampton, C. M., & Yazar-Klosinski, B. (2018). Ibogaine treatment outcomes for opioid dependence from a twelve-month follow-up observational study. *Am J Drug Alcohol Abuse, 44*(1), 37-46. doi:10.1080/00952990.2017.1310218
- Reiff, C. M., Richman, E. E., Nemeroff, C. B., Carpenter, L. L., Widge, A. S., Rodriguez, C. I., . . . McDonald, W. M. (2020). Psychedelics and Psychedelic-Assisted Psychotherapy. *Am J Psychiatry, 177*(5), 391-410. doi:10.1176/appi.ajp.2019.19010035
- Schenberg, E., Comis, M. A., Alexandre, J., Tófoli, L. F., Chaves, B., & Silveira, D. (2017). A phenomenological analysis of the subjective experience elicited by ibogaine in the context of a drug dependence treatment. *Journal of Psychedelic Studies, 1*, 1-10. doi:10.1556/2054.01.2017.007

ELEVEN
PSYCHEDELICS AND RELIGIOUS ORIGINS
SOPHIE SAINT THOMAS

Many of the psychedelics we use today, such as ayahuasca or peyote, were first used in religious ceremonies held by indigenous tribes. And contrary to popular belief and a dramatized perception of psychedelics as party drugs, it is the spiritual insight that is one of the most popular reasons to seek out psychedelic medicine. Today, there are people from all traditions and backgrounds within the psychedelic community. Keep in mind that the history of tribal use of psychedelic medicine for spiritual purposes is vast, and those interested in learning more about entheogens and indigenous cultures should seek out materials specifically relating to that topic.

LATIN AMERICAN RELIGIONS

Latin American countries have been using psychedelic medicine for millennia, and the trend is on the rise in modern society. Both the Aztecs and Maya in Central America used psychedelic medicine such as peyote and psilocybin mushrooms. Today, people flock to countries such as Brazil or Peru, where they can legally partake in ayahuasca retreats or experience San Pedro ceremonies.

While neither the Aztec nor Maya used ayahuasca, today, the brew, which is from the Amazon region of South America and made from two plants, is considered the most important holy plant medicine in Latin America. A 2019 study found that ayahuasca churches such as the "União de Vegetal" (UDV) group, a formal religion from Brazil that blends Christianity and traditional healing, have spread across the world (Estrella-Parra, Almanza-Pérez, & Alarcón-Aguilar, 2019). However, it is crucial to understand that the history of this region and entheogens is far vaster than one study can explain.

NATIVE AMERICAN RELIGIONS

The use of psychedelic plants and mushrooms was common among Native American tribes before the region was colonized. Psychedelics were used for both spiritual purposes and their healing properties. Like many indigenous cultures, they used plant medicines such as psilocybin mushrooms, peyote, and other less commonly known psychedelic plants to connect with ancestors and seek spiritual insight. Some historians believe that hallucinogens have been used as early as 9000 B.C. During colonization, plant medicine was quickly demonized — but not destroyed, thanks to unrelenting efforts by the Native American Church to protect and preserve their use of peyote as a sacrament. A 2019 study suggests that Native American youth today who identify with their culture are more likely to use peyote for spiritual purposes (Prince, O'Donnell, Stanley, & Swaim, 2019).

CHRISTIANITY

Because the U.S. has the largest Christian population in the world, at around 205 million as of 2015, it's impossible to apply a definitive statement on the modern use of psychedelics across the many diverse denominations of Christian faiths. While yes, some Christians take psychedelics, there is an interesting relationship between anti-drug propaganda, the rise of research limitations on psychedelics, and the moral imperative applied by vocal anti-drug leaders such as Ronald Reagan. Some historians, such as researchers Jerry B. Brown, Ph.D., and Julie M. Brown, authors of *The Psychedelic Gospels: The Secret History of Hallucinogens in Christianity,* go to great lengths to demonstrate the prevalence of psychedelics, in particular, psilocybin mushrooms, in Christian art. However, any past linkage may be Pagan in nature, as it is documented that Pagan traditions used entheogens (Winkelman, 2019). In *The Immortality Key: The Secret History of the Religion with No Name,* Brian C. Muraresku explores a potential psychedelic Eucharist for early Christians that evolved out of a tradition from Ancient Greece.

While Paganism was slightly tolerated in the early days of Christianity, it was outlawed during what's known as the "Constantine shift" between 313 to 391. However, many may have continued their tradition discretely and through a Christian lens. As psychedelics can help one understand their own holiness, spiritual revelations from a trip may even be considered blasphemous by some Christian-based faiths.

One notable moment in the history of Christianity and psychedelics is the 1962 Marsh Chapel Experiment, which took place during a Good Friday Service in Boston University's Marsh Chapel (Doblin, 1998). In a double-blind experiment, half of 20 divinity students were given psilocybin, while the control group received a large dose of niacin. Much of the experimental group experienced intense religious experiences. The findings suggest that psychedelics can encourage and enhance religious experiences.

JUDAISM

Like Christianity, Jewish thinkers have proposed that psychedelics could have played a role in early Judaism. A prominent theory is that the forbidden fruit eaten in the Garden of Eden was actually a psychedelic, which would certainly explain its role as a key to knowledge (Brown & Brown, 2019). Others theorize that manna, a divine fruit found by the Israelites in Exodus, could have been a psychoactive fungus (Shanon, 2008). Professor Benny Shanon of the Hebrew University of Jerusalem suggests that Moses' conversation with Yahweh and the bestowing of the Torah and meeting with the burning bush could have happened after he took DMT. "It seems logical that something was altered in people's consciousness," says Shanon. "There are other stories in the Bible that mention the use of plants: for example, the tree of the knowledge of good and evil in the Garden of Eden. The use of such substances, most of which fall in our contemporary Western culture under the label "drug," has in many traditions been considered sacred."

Modern-day psychedelic writers such as Madison Margolin have written prolifically about Judaism and psychedelics, in particular how they helped her reconnect with her Jewish identity. "I never felt so innately Jewish as when I did 5-MeO-DMT," Margolin writes in an essay titled "Returning Home: Jewish Trauma & Psychedelic Healing."

ISLAM

In Islam, the use of mind-altering substances is generally discouraged, as the Qur'an only references wine. In some Muslim countries, drug use can be met with the death penalty.

However, just like Jewish people or Christians, some modern Muslims do use psychedelic medicines, and it would be irresponsible to disclose them from any discussion on psychedelics and religion. In the book *Tripping with Allah: Islam, Drugs, and Writing*, Michael Muhammad Knight connects Islamic tradition with his experience drinking ayahuasca. His accessible personal narrative begins with him deciding to drink ayahuasca with the intention of having a visionary encounter with Fatima, the daughter of the Prophet Muhammad, and details how his experience brings him closer to Islam, leading to a change in his everyday habits.

HINDUISM

Unlike other popular modern religions, Hinduism has a solid relationship with psychedelics. The Vedas, or the first Hindu text, contain references and hymns devoted to Soma, a psychedelic drink. No one knows for sure what Soma was made out of, but it's believed to be psychedelic, likely from mushrooms (some even theorize that it grew in cow dung, which could be why cows are holy in Hinduism).

The Rigveda (8.48.3) reads, "We have drunk Soma and become immortal; we have attained the light, the Gods discovered. Now, what may foeman's malice do to harm us? What, O Immortal, mortal man's deception?" Hindu gods are often depicted in art with a cup of Soma in their hands. It's worth noting that Hinduism is accepting of cannabis, or ganja, in a way other religions are not. However, Hindu teachers do not see such substances as the key to enlightenment but as a powerful glimpse that must be coupled with work and dedication.

BUDDHISM

The biggest connection between psychedelics and Buddhism comes from pop culture, including many early psychedelic enthusiasts, such as Alan Watts, Aldous Huxley, Allen Ginsberg, and Ram Dass. Jack Kornfield once said that "LSD prepares the mind for Buddhism." But what about the original Buddhists, before Western psychedelic thinkers became turned on to the Four Noble Truths?

Although predominantly concerned with alcohol, the fifth precept is commonly quoted in favor of a sober Buddhist path. It reads, "I undertake the training rule to abstain from fermented drink that causes heedlessness." In *Secret Drugs of Buddhism: Psychedelic Sacraments and the Origins of the Vajrayana*, Michael Crowley writes of having studied Buddhist texts for decades and found repeated references to a substance called amrita, which translates to "deathless" or "nectar." According to Crowley, amrita was a psychoactive substance used in the Buddhist world during the Middle Ages. Crowley and other modern Buddhists agree that while psychedelic medicine is not incompatible with Buddhist teachings, one must also integrate meditation, study, and a mindful life if they are to use such substances to deepen their spiritual study.

CONCLUSION AND FINAL THOUGHTS

In many different religions throughout history, there have been reports of religious figures having mystical experiences that involved altered states of consciousness. So it is not surprising that some people today see psychedelics as a way to deepen their religious connection. Psychedelics can induce profound spiritual experiences, and when used with the proper guidance, they can be extremely beneficial. However, not all religions are equally open to the use of psychedelics. Native American religions and Buddhism, for example, have traditionally been more accepting of altered states of consciousness, and as a result, they fit much more easily into the psychedelic culture. Christianity and Islam, on the other hand, seem less compatible with psychedelic medicine at first glance. But there are individuals within these religions who are using psychedelics to enrich their spiritual lives.

Although we can continue to study the connections between religion and psychedelics, it is important for the psychedelic community not to make wide-scale judgments about any religion to ensure no one is excluded from the experience.

SUGGESTED FURTHER READINGS:

The Immortality Key: The Secret History of the Religion with No Name, by Brian C. Muraresku

DMT: The Spirit Molecule: A Doctor's Revolutionary Research into the Biology of Near-Death and Mystical Experiences, by Rick Strassman, MD

Entheogens and the Future of Religion, by Robert Forte

The Psychedelic Gospels: The Secret History of Hallucinogens in Christianity, by Jerry B. Brown, PhD and Julie M. Brown, MA

Secret Drugs of Buddhism: Psychedelic Sacraments and the Origins of the Vajrayana, by Michael Crowley and Ann Shulgin

Tripping with Allah: Islam, Drugs, and Writing, by Michael Muhammed Knight

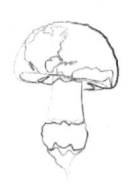

REFERENCES:

- Brown, J. B., & Brown, J. M. (2019). Entheogens in Christian art: Wasson, Allegro, and the Psychedelic Gospels. *Journal of Psychedelic Studies, 3*(2), 142-163. doi:10.1556/2054.2019.019
- Doblin, R. (1998). Dr. Leary's Concord Prison Experiment: a 34-year follow-up study. *J Psychoactive Drugs, 30*(4), 419-426. doi:10.1080/02791072.1998.10399715
- Estrella-Parra, E. A., Almanza-Pérez, J. C., & Alarcón-Aguilar, F. J. (2019). Ayahuasca: Uses, Phytochemical and Biological Activities. *Nat Prod Bioprospect, 9*(4), 251-265. doi:10.1007/s13659-019-0210-5
- Prince, M. A., O'Donnell, M. B., Stanley, L. R., & Swaim, R. C. (2019). Examination of Recreational and Spiritual Peyote Use Among American Indian Youth. *Journal of studies on alcohol and drugs, 80*(3), 366-370. doi:10.15288/jsad.2019.80.366
- Shanon, B. (2008). Biblical Entheogens: a Speculative Hypothesis. *Time and Mind, 1*(1), 51-74. doi:10.2752/175169608783489116
- Winkelman, M. (2019). Introduction: Evidence for entheogen use in prehistory and world religions. *Journal of Psychedelic Studies, 3*, 1-20. doi:10.1556/2054.2019.024

TWELVE
SEXUAL ABUSE IN PSYCHEDELIC CEREMONIES
LEIA FRIEDWOMAN, MS

Thank you to the dynamic array of people in psychedelic communities who are committed to ending sexual violence and who contributed to this article, including Katherine MacLean, Juliana Mulligan, Oriana Mayorga, Laura Mae Northrup, and Shea Prueger.

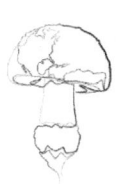

Sexual abuse is a complex and difficult topic, and there is no easy answer for how to address it. It can have devastating effects on individuals, families, and communities. It can cause physical and emotional damage, shatter trust, and undermine relationships. In the context of psychedelics, sexual abuse can occur when someone in a position of power takes advantage of their role to coerce or force sexual activity on another person. This can happen in a number of ways, including through manipulation, emotional manipulation, or physical force.

While sexual abuse can occur in any setting, it is especially harmful when it happens in a context where people are seeking healing and personal growth. To do this, we need to be open about the issue, educate ourselves about the prevalence and effects of sexual abuse, and develop policies and procedures that make it easier for survivors to come forward and get the help they need. This chapter will discuss sexual abuse in psychedelic ceremony contexts and what the community might do to better understand and prevent it. The article also includes some suggestions for how to address cases of sexual misconduct in psychedelic communities.

These matters can be challenging to read and think about. Please do what you need to do to take care of yourself. If you have experienced sexual harm in a psychedelic ceremony, you can visit www.psychedelic-survivors.com for support.

WHAT IS SEXUAL VIOLENCE?

Laura Mae Northrup, LMFT and host of Inside Eyes, a podcast about healing from sexual trauma with the use of psychedelics, defines sexual violence as a form of spiritual abuse. According to Northrup, "in the realm of psychology, we typically characterize sexual violence as an emotional, a psychological, or a physical form of abuse. In my opinion, it is all of those things. It's a form of abuse that enacts violence on the very core of one's vitality, meaning, their sexuality. And while spirituality can be hard to define from a scientific perspective, from a felt sense perspective, any violence that attacks sexuality is an attack on the human spirit and, in its wake, leaves a spiritual wound. I would argue that sexual violence crushes the human spirit."

Sexual violence is a serious and pervasive problem in our society. One in four women will be sexually assaulted at some point in their lives, and approximately one in six men. Nonbinary and transgender individuals are often at even greater risk of experiencing assault and abuse than cisgender people. Sexual violence can take many forms, from unwanted touching to actual or attempted unwanted penetration by an object or body part, denying a person contraception or protection against sexually transmitted diseases, taking any kind of sexual pictures or film without a person's consent, forcing a person to perform sexual acts, threatening to break up with or hurt a person if they refuse sex, and more. It is an act of power and control, not one of love.

Sexual violence can have a far-reaching negative effect on people. Exposure to sexual violence is outlined in the DSM-5 criteria for PTSD. Victims of sexual violence often suffer from long-term physical and mental health problems, such as depression, anxiety, and post-traumatic stress disorder. They may also have difficulty trusting others and forming healthy relationships.

It is important to remember that sexual violence is never the victim's fault. All sexual exchanges should be consensual: a voluntary agreement made without coercion between persons with decision-making capacity, knowledge, understanding, and autonomy. Consent is freely given, reversible, informed, enthusiastic, and specific. The Art of Giving and Receiving is a great book for anyone wanting to take a deep dive into the topic of consent.

There should be no pressure, force, manipulation, or intoxication involved in obtaining consent. In the case of a psychedelic ceremony, due to the nature of the psychedelic experience, a person cannot consent to sex because they are in an altered state of consciousness. Even if a sexual advance is made not during the ceremony but before or after, consent is still tricky to navigate. A person may be deep in their own process, vulnerable, and dealing with a lot, rendering their decision-making capacity limited. The time leading up to a psychedelic ceremony or retreat and the time afterward is an altered state of its own.

A facilitator with integrity will understand the power dynamics inherent in the healing relationship and not pursue adding a dual dimension of romantic or sexual intimacy. It is a violation of healer and religious/spiritual codes of conduct for someone who is providing medicine to engage in sexual relations with their clients/ceremony attendees. While it is not necessarily guaranteed to be harmful in every single instance, the potential for harm is significant and must not be ignored.

People can be more open or "receptive" after a psychedelic journey, and it is a facilitator's responsibility to help (or at least not hurt) the person as they go through their experience. If someone is experiencing a sexual awakening or a reclaiming of sexual power, it is sexual violence for the facilitator to take advantage of that. There is an intrinsic power dynamic that the practitioner holds, especially in situations where the healer has a following, similar to a guru.

WHAT ARE POWER DYNAMICS?

Power dynamics are the relationships between people in which one person has more power than the other. Power is present in social, political, and economic contexts and confers to those who hold it more ability to make decisions, take action, or even avoid negative consequences. It is often said that "power corrupts, and absolute power corrupts absolutely." This adage suggests that power dynamics are inherently dangerous and that those who hold power are more likely to abuse it. However, it is important to remember that power is not necessarily a bad thing. Like a knife, power can be wielded in service of help or harm.

In order to understand power, we must first recognize it. We live in a society with systemic injustice, including white supremacy, colonialism, patriarchy, ableism, cis/heterosexism, transphobia, and more. This society confers more power to people who fit into the dominant paradigm. Regrettably, psychedelic communities are not immune to these power imbalances.

In a 2018 event entitled <u>Male Supremacy and the Psychedelic Patriarchy</u>, Katherine MacLean, Ph.D. shared that "nearly all of the world's psychedelic research groups and funding organizations are led by cis white men, even though women and people of color make up more than half of the clinicians, research staff, volunteers, and visionaries fueling and guiding these institutions." Many psychedelic conferences, community groups, and venues are likewise headlined, organized, and led by men, even though women and gender non-conforming individuals make up a large segment of the attendees, public speakers, and social activists.

It is still unclear who will have access to psychedelic therapies; considering the US's racial disparities, health disparities, healthcare crisis, and exorbitant wealth stratification, psychedelic therapy could simply become a thing only accessible to privileged, mostly white populations. Although psychedelic populations tout unity and oneness, power is not evenly distributed in our psychedelic spaces. Most organizations still employ hierarchical structures, and power dynamics often go unrecognized.

In a psychedelic ceremony, the facilitator or shaman has power because of their position. The Chacruna Institute's Ayahuasca Community Guidelines for the Awareness of Sexual Abuse says that "'shamans are often highly romanticized in the Western imagination. Some South American and indeed Western men have learned to take advantage of exalted images of healers."

Power is not held as a binary, where people either have it or don't have it. Many people have intersecting identities, and so they may have power in some ways but not in others. For instance, a South American shaman may hold power because of their position as a healer, providing what some would call life-saving services. Participants have compensated this person for their services. If they are a man, society confers power to them (the Shipibo people have a matriarchal society, so they may be an exception). On the other hand, a ceremony participant with light skin, access to financial resources, and other forms of privilege may hold power that a South American shaman does not.

The dynamics of a facilitator and participant are complex. There may be feelings of emotional intimacy of varying intensities that arise, and it is the facilitator's responsibility to make sure the participant is safe, and those boundaries are kept.

Due to the lack of regulation and licensing with most psychedelics, there is often no system of accountability for the facilitator to answer to. This is one of several factors that further complicate addressing and preventing sexual abuse in psychedelic ceremonies.

THE PREVALENCE OF SEXUAL VIOLENCE IN PSYCHEDELIC CEREMONIES

Although it is often shrouded in secrecy and shame, sexual violence is a pervasive problem in our society, even in medical and psychotherapy settings. There is no single explanation for why people engage in sexual violence. Some people may do it out of a sense of power or entitlement, while others may be acting out of anger or resentment. Some perpetrators may have underlying mental health issues, such as psychosis or personality disorders. Others may have been sexually abused themselves. Still, others may simply see sex as something they are entitled to, or as a way to control or dominate others. This is by no means an exhaustive explanation, although it may provide a framework for a better understanding of such cases.

Cultural norms impact different understandings of sexual abuse in ritual contexts and the ways people respond to survivors, perpetrators, and the general public after a violation has occurred. Rape culture is defined as "stereotyped, false beliefs about rape that justify sexual aggression and trivialize the seriousness of sexual violence." Rape culture perpetuates the belief that a survivor of sexual violence is responsible for or contributed to their victimization.

A frightening element of rape culture is that people are taught how to try to *avoid* being raped rather than how to *avoid raping*. Living in a society with a rape culture contributes to the harm of sexual violence to the victim and community. To make matters even more complex, people who enact sexual violence typically have their own issues with substance use, emotional trauma, depression, anxiety, or even a history of being abused themselves (Glasser et al., 2001).

In a study of survivors of childhood sexual abuse (CSA), researchers found that women who had experienced CSA were more likely to be sexually victimized as adults, while men who experienced CSA were more likely to become perpetrators of sexual abuse as adults (Hailes, Yu, Danese, & Fazel, 2019). It is important to note that sexual violence affects all genders, and 2SLGBTQIA+ people are as likely or more likely to experience sexual violation than cis-gendered or straight individuals (Martin-Storey et al., 2018). Sexual violence can happen to any gender or be enacted by any gender. Women, trans people, and people of color are most likely to experience this form of trauma.

Another factor that can lead to sexual violence is when facilitators are not trained to handle transference. Transference is a psychological concept when a person projects or displaces feelings for someone in their life onto their therapist or healer. Feeling sexually or romantically attracted to a facilitator can be a form of transference, as can relating to a facilitator as though they are a parent, friend, partner, or family member. A facilitator or shaman who is not getting their needs met in their life may seek to fulfill their desire with the vulnerable people attending the ceremony by taking advantage of transference, especially if a participant is projecting sexual feelings onto the facilitator as part of their healing process.

Juliana Mulligan, an ibogaine integration specialist and co-founder of The Root Ibogaine Collective, uses the term "shaman complex" to describe people who escape a feeling of low self-esteem by becoming exalted healers.

"Stepping into the role of 'healer' is perfect for anyone with sociopathic or personality disorder traits; you get to have the power of others, receive admiration, potentially claim that you're some kind of prodigy, and actually make money from all of this," she said in an article on Chacruna (Mulligan, 2020). Mulligan also describes how psychological abuse and manipulation are another concerning force in psychedelic ceremony spaces.

Shea Prueger, director of Ibogaine Revelations, talks about cases of blurred boundaries she has seen in psychedelic ceremony communities. "Remote and communal living have remained popular among psychedelic enthusiasts. There are communities that tend to grow and exist around a shaman or a team of medicine facilitators, and in these cases, frequent ceremony participants might choose - or be asked - to live on the land where the ceremonies are held. Some people might pay money for a room, while others might work out a deal for a "work trade." People in this situation are easily taken advantage of and are also vulnerable to the expectations of the community, which can center around romanticizing a central or head figure.

As people may live in these communities for months or even years, the roles of who is a participant and who is a friend or family member are easily blurred, or individuals can feel pressure to act a certain way to keep in good standing within the community. Sometimes these communities are overseas; they often attract younger individuals, oftentimes women, who may pay money to stay or not have other means to leave once they are there and committed to a communal situation. This leads to an extremely vulnerable situation, especially if the facilitator is taking advantage of boundaries and their respect and admiration in a community."

A person attending a psychedelic ceremony is in a vulnerable state. During the ceremony, they are in the care of the facilitator(s) and staff and should be treated with consideration, care, and respect at all times. Considering that some people may be coming to a psychedelic ceremony to *heal* from sexual trauma, it is especially concerning to think that someone could be sexually abused during a psychedelic ceremony. For those looking to heal sexual trauma in a psychedelic ceremony, adding in a trauma-informed therapist or practitioner with training on sexual trauma resolution could help in the overall experience. The practitioner can help provide preliminary processing before the ceremony and integration support and continued processing after the ceremony.

There are numerous anecdotal reports of ayahuasca shamans who intentionally seek out sexual relations with participants.

Sexual exploitation in iboga and ibogaine ceremonies is also common. "There have been allegations of ibogaine providers engaging in sexual relationships with clients, often using their position of power or as a "healer" to get what they want," says Prueger.

Unfortunately, no research has been conducted to date on how prevalent sexual abuse is in psychedelic ceremonies. There is no regulatory body or certification that facilitators of psychedelic ceremonies are beholden to, and the underground/secret nature of many psychedelic ceremonies can contribute further to the lack of accountability.

PREVENTING SEXUAL VIOLENCE IN PSYCHEDELIC CEREMONIES

Screening participants can rule out individuals who may not be safe. Ceremony holders should uphold a culture of consent and respect other people's boundaries, and know their own. Practitioners should be trauma-informed, deeply committed to ethics and right-relationship, aware of power dynamics, and should act accordingly. Psychedelic ceremony leaders should understand that rape culture exists and seek to interrupt it.

Prueger advises that psychedelic facilitators create a mutual consent contract that would be presented during a participant's intake process. "A mutual consent contract can re-inform boundaries and what is expected from each person during someone's process, and re-define roles between participant, facilitator, and various staff members. It will let a participant know what sort of behavior is expected from everyone involved in their process."

Facilitators should be responsible for their own self-care and the continuation of their own healing. "It is particularly common with ibogaine for facilitators to sprout up shortly after their first session with the medicine," Prueger says. "Many people are enthusiastic about the medicine and genuinely want to spread their experience to others. However, while some of these people may have broken away from their substance dependency and feel healed, they may now have a host of trauma and other behaviors that deserve time, attention, and continued therapy or care -- but are now in the position of taking care of others. Normalizing the idea that practitioners should be in therapy, continuing their education and training, and working on themselves may build better and safer practitioners."

If a psychedelic ceremony leader or staff has violated a participant, they should not be allowed around people in vulnerable states. A trauma-informed approach is important, as these ruptures in the community can easily lead to compounded harm for survivors and the community at large.

If someone has been harmed or violated in an underground setting, they may benefit from processing the experience with a licensed, trauma-informed therapist. They may find a level of safety in the confidential communication and boundaried relationship between therapist and client. Talking to a therapist outside of the psychedelic community could provide an objective third party for the client to process with, although some survivors of sexual abuse in psychedelic ceremonies have expressed difficulty with therapists and family members bringing the perspective that psychedelic ceremonies are not safe. Knowledge and respect for nuance is important, as a therapy license does not automatically mean that the person understands the complex ins and outs of the psychedelic sector.

For some people, processing a violation feels more supportive in the context of peer support, such as with other survivors of psychedelic ceremony/therapy abuse.

Harmed parties should be consulted and taken into consideration every step of the way as the community decides how to address the incident. The community should come together, and those who feel called can help support survivors while others offer accountability support to people who caused harm. Psychedelic communities can uphold accountability by practicing it in our personal lives and modeling this behavior of integrity and self-responsibility in our interactions and relationships.

Mulligan also suggests that the staff at ceremonies or clinics should be comprised of at least half women and/or non-binary individuals. "The leadership of the ceremony or treatment center should not be exclusively male either; this should also be a minimum of 50% individuals who are not cis-men. Understanding and being sensitive to the trauma that women and non-binary people experience requires specialized training that most men in this industry just don't have."

DEMANDING ACCOUNTABILITY

If a person can recognize the harm that they have caused to another person and, by extension, the community, they may want to repair the harm. These are complex processes that are best held in the hands of experienced facilitators. Recognizing the problem and actively participating in treatment and recovery may reduce the likelihood that someone will commit more sexual harm.

It is critical to consider whether a restorative or transformative justice process should take place if it is at the expense of or further detriment to any harmed party. Careful consideration must be given to those who have experienced harm, as well as those who might be harmed in any process.

"Some transformative processes that we've seen in psychedelic communities around sexual violence have failed, or at least fallen short of achieving meaningful transformation and collective healing," says Oriana Mayorga, Board Director at SSDP and SPORE. Mayorga organized one of the first series around sexual violence, Psychedelic Sisters in Arms, in 2018. "That doesn't mean that we shouldn't move toward community accountability as a method to deal with these situations."

Restorative and transformative justice is a technology that has been stewarded by indigenous cultures, such as the Māori of New Zealand and First Nations people in Canada, for a long time. Black communities and disabled communities of color have also utilized restorative justice to uphold safety, as law enforcement was not safe for them to trust. Restorative justice processes are best held in the hands of experienced facilitators and with transparency for the community.

COMING TOGETHER TO END SEXUAL VIOLENCE IN PSYCHEDELIC CEREMONIES

As responsible members of society, it is incumbent upon each of us to play our part in recognizing, addressing, and eliminating sexual violence. This is no less true for those who facilitate psychedelic ceremonies, and who have a duty of care to keep participants safe from harm. In the event that sexual misconduct does occur, we must be mindful of not further traumatizing those who have already been harmed. This means listening to survivors without judgment, respecting their wishes and boundaries, and taking steps to ensure their safety and well-being.

Restorative and transformative justice are potential avenues for exploration as psychedelic communities contend with how to help people who have caused harm and want to be accountable. Restorative justice does not work in a punitive sense and will not work well if it is forced; the person must *want* to change.

For immediate support regarding sexual violence, call 800-656-HOPE to speak with someone from RAINN (Rape, Assault, and Incest National Network).

To speak to someone about concerns relating to these matters in psychedelic communities, visit www.psychedelic-survivors.com.

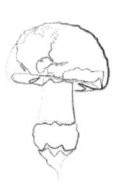

REFERENCES:

- Glasser, M., Kolvin, I., Campbell, D., Glasser, A., Leitch, I., & Farrelly, S. (2001). Cycle of child sexual abuse: Links between being a victim and becoming a perpetrator. *British Journal of Psychiatry, 179*(6), 482-494. doi:10.1192/bjp.179.6.482
- Hailes, H. P., Yu, R., Danese, A., & Fazel, S. (2019). Long-term outcomes of childhood sexual abuse: an umbrella review. *Lancet Psychiatry, 6*(10), 830-839. doi:10.1016/s2215-0366(19)30286-x
- Martin-Storey, A., Paquette, G., Bergeron, M., Dion, J., Daigneault, I., Hébert, M., & Ricci, S. (2018). Sexual Violence on Campus: Differences Across Gender and

Sexual Minority Status. *Journal of Adolescent Health, 62*(6), 701-707. doi:https://doi.org/10.1016/j.jadohealth.2017.12.013
- Mulligan, J. (2020). Abuses and Lack of Safety in the Ibogaine Community. *Chacruna*. Retrieved from https://chacruna.net/ibogaine-abuses-accountability/

THIRTEEN
PSYCHEDELICS AND THE CONTROLLED SUBSTANCES ACT
KATIE STONE, MA

Imagine this snapshot in U.S. history. The year is 1969. Psychedelic drugs have become popular among young people as a way of exploring consciousness, community, and reality. The Vietnam War rages on with no end in sight. College students are out protesting and demanding peace, citizens are refusing the draft, and members of the armed forces have come back from service carrying painful wounds and memories of the events they witnessed. The Civil Rights Movement, the Environmental Movement, the Anti-War Movement, the American Indian Movement, and the Feminist Movement are all underway, and social order seems entirely uncertain.

Amid this social climate, and under President Nixon's administration in the early 70s, the United States mounts an aggressive campaign to win back public opinion in America, all while simultaneously criminalizing his opposition. The plan calls for hitting countercultural youth and communities of color - those who oppose his policies the loudest- with a War on Drugs that continues today.

THE CONTROLLED SUBSTANCES ACT

The Controlled Substances Act (CSA) was passed in 1970. The law made it a federal crime to manufacture, distribute, or possess many drugs, and it imposed stiff penalties for those who violated the law. The CSA was controversial from the start, and critics argue that the law is ineffective and unfairly punishes people who use drugs. Rather than prioritizing social support, the CSA opened the door for the militarization of the police and racial profiling in policing.

With this legislation, Nixon launched the War on Drugs against the 1960s counterculture movement. But it was not just a war against LSD and the anti-war movement; it was also against the Civil Rights Movement. Admittedly, says Nixon's aide John Ehrlichman:

"We knew we couldn't make it illegal to be either against the war or black, but by getting the public to associate the hippies with marijuana and blacks with heroin. And then, criminalizing both heavily, we could disrupt those communities. We could arrest their leaders, raid their homes, break up their meetings, and vilify them night after night on the evening news. Did we know we were lying about the drugs? Of course we did."

Prior to this overarching law, drug laws were a patchwork of legislation. LSD, for example, was illegal to sell or manufacture thanks to 1966 legislation, but it was the CSA that made possession of psychedelics a federal offense. Before its passage, psychedelic drugs like LSD were widely used among students and young people, as well as cultural leaders and other members of society who wanted to explore alternative ways of experiencing reality. They were also used by therapists in clinical practice and had been researched clinically for decades and used successfully in mental health treatment.

However, the passage of the Controlled Substances Act, which classified psychedelic drugs as Schedule I substances with no medical value and a high potential for abuse or addiction, would change all that.

The CSA was passed in 1970, and it classified drugs into five categories or schedules. Schedule I substances are considered to have a high potential for abuse, have no currently accepted medical use (in the United States), and are unsafe to use even if under supervision by healthcare professionals. Schedules II-V include progressively less harmful drugs and are regulated based on their potential to be abused without a doctor's supervision (Schedule V is considered non-addictive).

But the Nixon administration was less worried about public health and more concerned about public opposition to the Vietnam War and the growing public support for civil rights.

A RACIST DRUG WAR

The U.S.-led war on drugs began when federal funding was funneled toward its infrastructure, but it was not the first drug law passed among states or municipalities. Rather, it was preceded by other laws that explicitly targeted minority groups.

For example, the oldest drug law - passed in 1875 - was explicitly aimed at Chinese communities. In the early 20th century, cocaine and marijuana laws were also accompanied by racist propaganda that stoked social tensions and ignored the traditional and medicinal uses. None of these laws were motivated entirely by public health concerns; all were accompanied by a desire to oppress minority groups through the implementation of policies that attack culturally relevant drugs and medicines.

In 1914, Congress passed the Harrison Narcotics Act, which prohibited any non-medical use of cocaine and opium without first obtaining an expensive prescription from licensed doctors — this effectively criminalized communities where these drugs had been used for years as part of traditional medical care. Such a policy impacted social groups at very different rates.

In 1924, when the prohibition of alcohol and its accompanying moral panic period was underway, Congress passed the Anti-Heroin Act and outlawed the importation and possession of opium for manufacturing heroin. This was an amendment to the 1909 Smoking Opium Exclusion Act that targeted Chinese communities, where opium has been used medicinally for millennia. These punitive types of drug war tactics continued throughout the 20th century until Nixon's presidency escalated exponentially by making psychedelic substances such as LSD Schedule I drugs.

Today, despite hard-fought reforms that have reduced some of the worst excesses of the War on Drugs, communities continue to be disproportionately impacted by drug laws along the lines of race, gender, and social class.

ENDING THE WAR ON DRUGS

Current drug laws are based on the belief that certain types of drug use should always be criminalized, while other types of drug use can be socially acceptable. Such framings do not reflect the latest evidence-based research on addiction theory or harm-reduction approaches to drug misuse.

Furthermore, the War on Drugs has failed to eliminate drug use or improve public safety. It has instead caused immense harm to communities and families and contributed to mass incarceration. Given this history, it is clear that the current legal situation does not readily support people experiencing chaotic drug use of any kind, nor does it lay a solid foundation for future psychedelic therapy models.

When President Nixon passed the Controlled Substances Act in 1970, the ranked level of drug scheduling determined the corresponding level of a criminal conviction. Punishments ranged from fines, incarceration, and even forcible rehab, often at contracted facilities that are notorious for safety and ethics violations. Mandatory minimum sentencing was enacted, prison populations grew rapidly, and amendments to the CSA and various crime bills have all continued to build evermore jail cells. At the same time, a private prison industry took hold during the Regan and Clinton administrations, with great support from now-President Biden.

Today, the United States is the most heavily incarcerated nation, with Black men and their families bearing the brunt of police targeting. In a drug war where rates of use are similar, Black Americans are 2.7 times more likely to be arrested for drug-related offenses. Just as young people and students were demanding an end to the Vietnam War 50 years ago, they are now demanding an end to the drug war — not just for psychedelics but also for all drugs.

Oregon was the first state to decriminalize drug possession in 2020, dropping the crime from a criminal offense to a reduced fine, a move that Kassandra Frederique, Executive Director of the Drug Policy Alliance, called the first domino to fall in the "cruel and inhumane war on drugs." That same election, Oregon passed a measure to develop a psilocybin-assisted therapy program. These measures were passed simultaneously, not through a unified campaign, and because these are only state laws, federal laws still technically apply.

Even after psychedelic therapy is legalized, this form of healing will only be available to people who have access to licensed healthcare — many people will continue to seek psychedelics through underground markets and healers. Of these, many will still be brought into the criminal justice system. But only if these prohibitive drug laws are still in place. Addressing mandatory minimum sentencing, bail, family separation, asset forfeiture, and other prominent issues in the criminal justice system will help, but ultimately, an entirely different approach to drugs is necessary at the federal level.

Part of healing the mental health crisis in the United States includes addressing the sources of trauma and suffering that perpetuate cycles of chaotic drug use. It also involves addressing the harms and failures caused by the fifty-year-old war on drugs and holding conversations about how we as a society will choose to navigate potential dangers and personal liberty going forward.

The criminal justice system is one of the biggest sources of violence in U.S. society, and it disproportionately targets people of color and low-income people. Ending the immediate harm caused by the War on Drugs is essential and will allow room for exploring alternatively scheduling strategies, designing better-informed research studies, and developing evidence-based social support programs that are truly intended to support public health, rather than to oppress or criminalize certain social groups.

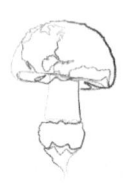

FOURTEEN
PSYCHEDELIC HARM REDUCTION STRATEGIES AND STUDIES
MARGARET SHARPE, MSW, LCSW

Since its inception, harm reduction has been a controversial topic. Some people feel that it condones illegal behavior, while others believe it is a more realistic and practical approach than complete abstinence. The goal of harm reduction is not to judgmentally dictate what people should or should not do, but rather to provide resources and information so that people can make informed choices about their behaviors. It is built on the belief that people have the right to make their own decisions about their lives, even if those decisions may be harmful. While harm reduction does not condone illegal behaviors, it does acknowledge that they will occur and seeks to minimize their impact. This approach has been shown to be effective in reducing the spread of disease, lowering drug-related death rates, and decreasing overall crime rates. In many ways, harm reduction is a more compassionate and realistic approach than complete abstinence. Rather than condemning people for their choices, harm reduction offers them a way to improve their quality of life.

Harm reduction was developed as a reaction to the legalistic system that dominated laws, especially since the US Controlled Substance Act of 1970, which many countries worldwide still take their cues from. The first model of this nature, the Mersey Harm Reduction Model, was developed in the mid-1980s in Liverpool, England (O'Hare, 2007). Rather than pushing an abstinence-only model, the model focused on reducing harms related to drug use, particularly with heroin injection. The initial goal was to reduce the transmission of HIV, but the blueprint transferred well when MDMA use took off.

The National Harm Reduction Coalition describes this modality as "a set of practical strategies and ideas aimed at reducing negative consequences associated with drug use. Harm reduction is also a movement for social justice built on a belief in, and respect for, the rights of people who use drugs." The goal is to minimize the negative effects of drug use rather than condemn or further isolate people who use drugs

Harm reduction includes educational campaigns and care provided at health facilities. One well-known harm reduction policy is the implementation of needle exchange programs for people who inject heroin. By providing clean needles and other sanitary drug paraphernalia such as alcohol pads, sets of micron-filters, and "cookers," the risk of transmitting communicable diseases such as HIV and hepatitis is reduced. Additionally, these services often provide Narcan (a pharmaceutical for reversing an opiate overdose) and fentanyl drug tests, which reduce the risk of bodily harm and death. Other well-known harm reduction programs include methadone clinics and "safer sex" programs in schools.

The Drug Policy Alliance is an organization that advocates for an end to the War on Drugs. They believe that the current policies and attitudes towards drugs are causing more harm than good, and they are working to promote policies that will offset the harms of drug use and prohibition. One of the ways they are doing this is by supporting the sovereignty of the individual to make decisions about their own mind and body.

STUDIES RELATED TO PSYCHEDELICS AND HARM REDUCTION STRATEGIES

Though most psychedelics remain illegal, it's estimated that over thirty million people in the US have used them at least once in their lifetime (Krebs & Johansen, 2013). People are increasingly seeking out these psychoactive substances for the treatment of mental health conditions, especially as research and decriminalization efforts have increased in recent years.

So how do psychedelics fit into this paradigm? Those that are produced in labs (like Lysergic acid diethylamide, or LSD, dissociatives (like ketamine) and dextromethorphan, or DXM), and other entheogens (like MDMA), are all important to include in the harm reduction model due to the risks involved with their use. Testing, education, and supportive services, particularly at music events and "transformational" festivals (like Burning Man), have been shown to be incredibly beneficial. Many of these events have water stations, "chill" spaces or "challenging trip" tents, test kits, medical staff, and other supportive services available on site.

Educational websites, such as Erowid.com and TheGoodDrugGuide.com, among others, are non-profits committed to providing information to the public about psychoactive substances. Erowid includes basic information about the substance, history, effects, health impacts, legal status, dosage information, chemistry, as well as personal accounts and "trip reports."

The Zendo Project is a well-known organization focusing on this model. Its mission is to provide education, resources, guidance, and support, particularly at events where people are more likely to use psychedelics, like festivals and concerts. Zendo volunteers are trained to provide high-quality, non-judgmental, trauma-informed support to reduce the number of hospitalizations and psychiatric arrests. The psychological support of helping someone through a "bad trip" can be invaluable. A bad trip is often caused by a lack of preparation or lack of attention to set (mindset before the trip), setting (location and company kept), and an inappropriate dose of the drug (too much or too little).

With harm reduction services that provide psychological support, a "bad" trip may be approached as "difficult" instead, with potential for growth. Although it may not be easy to go through, a difficult experience can yield profound realizations and even be incredibly transformative for a person. This could be the difference between involuntary psychiatric intervention while in a vulnerable state and trauma-informed care that may be deeply valuable to a person later.

Zendo also provides education and resources on its website to help people prepare ahead of time for safer use. There are other organizations, like Dancewize in Australia, that provide similar services.

Test kits allow people to test the content and purity of their substances before consumption. Test kits may encourage someone to use less by specifying dosing amounts and helping people avoid dangerous additives or combinations. Due to the drug's popularity, the first test kits focused on MDMA, which is often adulterated with other substances that mimic its effects but can be more dangerous.

The most well-known source of test kits in the US is DanceSafe, which also sells rapid result kits for LSD, ketamine, MDMA, and more. The most accurate MDMA test is chromatography/mass spectrometry (GC/MS) and is offered by Erowid. There are other test kits sold on the internet, such as BunkPolice.

Potentially dangerous additives such as fentanyl, cathinones ("bath salts"), methamphetamine, PMA, PMMA, and 25i-NBOMe can be detected with these kits. Unfortunately, test kits are considered drug paraphernalia and may be confiscated in festival settings, which can be a deterrent.

Websites like Rollsafe.org provide comprehensive education, safety/risk considerations, and guidance regarding reducing the potentially harmful effects of MDMA. This includes research-based neuroprotective supplement recommendations. Rollsafe donates a high percentage of its proceeds to the Multidisciplinary Association for Psychedelic Studies (MAPS), a non-profit organization that has dedicated over thirty years to researching the therapeutic use of MDMA.

Psychedelic integration therapy is another framework that looks at ways to reduce risk and harm in the immediate days after a trip and promotes the long-term well-being of the individual. Although there are ethical and legal considerations to providing this kind of support to clients, it is important that therapists are educated in this model and aware their clients may be interested in psychedelic medicine. To find a psychedelic integration practitioner in your area, consult Psychable.com, MAPS.org, Tripsitters.org, or Psychedelics.support.

PSYCHEDELIC HARM REDUCTION: SHIFTING POWER INTO THE HANDS OF THE INDIVIDUAL

Psychedelics have been used for centuries by indigenous cultures for healing and spiritual purposes. In recent years, there has been a resurgence of interest in these substances, as well as a growing body of scientific evidence supporting their safety and efficacy.

Psychedelics can create profound shifts in states of consciousness, and the psychedelic harm reduction model does not attempt to minimize or ignore the harms and dangers of illicit drug use. Rather, it puts the power into the hands of the individual to make more well-informed choices about their use. Harm reduction is a more humane way to approach human behavior. This model stands for drug policies that are therapeutic rather than punitive. It advocates for human rights and humanity, in general; harm reduction is re-humanizing.

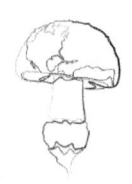

REFERENCES:

- Krebs, T. S., & Johansen, P. (2013). Over 30 million psychedelic users in the United States. *F1000Res, 2*, 98. doi:10.12688/f1000research.2-98.v1
- O'Hare, P. (2007). Merseyside, the first harm reduction conferences, and the early history of harm reduction. *International Journal of Drug Policy, 18*(2), 141-144. doi:https://doi.org/10.1016/j.drugpo.2007.01.003

PART THREE
KETAMINE

(The discovery of the effects of ketamine on depression are)
"arguably the most important discovery in half a century."

Science Magazine

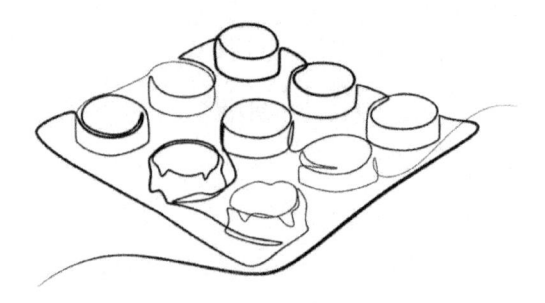

FIFTEEN
A BEGINNER'S GUIDE TO KETAMINE
SOPHIE SAINT THOMAS

MEDICALLY REVIEWED BY DR. DAVID FLYNN, MD, MBA, CPHQ

Ketamine was first used as an anesthetic on the battlefields of Vietnam and later became popular in the club kid rave scene. Today, ketamine is being used as a treatment for those experiencing treatment-resistant depression, PTSD, suicidal thoughts, and several other conditions. While colloquially called a psychedelic, ketamine is technically a dissociative anesthetic and is still used in operating rooms and ERs across the country. Some argue that ketamine is a life-saving drug that offers hope to those who have exhausted all other options. Others claim that ketamine is dangerous and addictive, with long-term effects that are not yet fully understood. This chapter presents the facts so that you can make your own informed decision.

WHAT IS KETAMINE?

Ketamine is a dissociative anesthetic with psychedelic properties. It was discovered in 1956 and approved in 1970 as an anesthetic agent derived from phencyclidine. Unlike most anesthetics, ketamine maintains hemodynamic stability, or stable blood flow, which is crucial when treating trauma patients. It's listed on the World Health Organization Model List of Essential Medicines, which names medications considered to be most effective and safe while meeting a health system's most important needs.

Ketamine is also used as an alternative to opiate pain-relievers. With more than 20,000 published reports detailing ketamine's biological safety over the past 50 years and many reports on its effectiveness with mental health dating back to 1974, ketamine is emerging as a novel treatment for depression, PTSD, suicidal thoughts, and other mental health conditions. It is currently the only legal psychedelic drug in the United States. Ketamine is also used as a recreational drug due to its hallucinogenic and dissociative effects.

WHAT IS KETAMINE USED TO TREAT?

While ketamine was originally used as an anesthetic, it is now also used off-label to treat depression, PTSD, anxiety, and other conditions. While it's not the first line of treatment, a growing body of research suggests it can be beneficial for those experiencing depression and other mental health conditions who do not respond to traditional antidepressants such as SSRIs or those who prefer not to take a daily medication. Ketamine also has a favorable side effect profile when used appropriately. Below are the primary indications for ketamine.

Medical and Surgical Use

Although it's often referred to as a psychedelic, ketamine is technically a cyclohexanone derivative with analgesic and anesthetic properties. While more research is needed to fully understand its mechanism of action, evidence suggests that ketamine works by exerting complex pharmacological actions, including inhibition of biogenic amine uptake, binding to opioid receptors, and inhibition of N-methyl D-aspartate (NMDA) receptors.

Ketamine is an exceptionally useful anesthetic because, unlike other anesthetics, it is unlikely to cause reductions in blood pressure, breathing, or loss of airway reflexes. Due it its relative safety, it has long been used in pediatric and veterinary medicine for pain control, sedation, and anesthesia. More recently, ketamine has become very popular in patients of all ages during surgery because it reduces the need for opioid pain relievers after surgery.

Depression

At subanesthetic doses, ketamine can be effective as a treatment for depression. Research suggests that ketamine can provide rapid relief to people with treatment-resistant depression. It is estimated that 10-30% of people with depression are resistant to the beneficial effects of traditional antidepressants (Bystritsky, 2006). Even for those who do respond, antidepressants such as SSRIs can take weeks to take effect and have challenging side effects (Garakani et al., 2020). Because ketamine treatment can show results in a matter of hours after administration, it is particularly useful for patients experiencing suicidal thoughts or ideation (D'Anci, Uhl, Giradi, & Martin, 2019). There is also evidence supporting its use for bipolar depression (Zanos & Gould, 2018).

While the most noted ketamine studies for depression were done off-label using intravenous infusions, in 2019, a nasal spray called Spravato (esketamine) was approved for use by the Food and Drug Administration (FDA). Recently, several studies have also been done showing the effectiveness of oral ketamine for depression and symptoms of anxiety (Domany et al., 2018; Dore et al., 2019; Glue et al., 2020; Irwin et al., 2013).

Anxiety

While most of the mental health research on ketamine relates to depression, with which anxiety is often a comorbid condition, there are indications that ketamine may help treat anxiety as well. Multiple studies on people with symptoms of anxiety or a diagnosed anxiety disorder found that ketamine resulted in a significantly greater reduction in anxiety relative to placebo. One recent retrospective review looked at the impact of oral ketamine combined with psychotherapy on anxiety symptoms of 235 patients across three private practices over a five-year period (Dore et al., 2019). Anxiety scores fell an average of 5.5 points, going from moderate to mild during treatment. Treatment duration showed that the longer the duration of treatment, the greater the improvement in anxiety. More research directly pertaining to anxiety disorders and symptoms is needed.

PTSD

Much like depression, the current treatments available for PTSD, such as SSRIs, have limited efficacy. As a result, ketamine is increasingly being used by people experiencing post-traumatic stress disorder.

In a 2021 study, patients received either ketamine or a placebo six times over two weeks. The results suggest that ketamine infusions reduced symptoms in chronic PTSD patients. Of the ketamine patients, 67% experienced symptom relief, compared with 20% in the placebo group (Feder et al., 2021). The result lasted a median of 27.5 days, suggesting the use of booster infusions to maintain results. For patients who receive ketamine infusions, the typical treatment protocol can be an initial six rounds of treatment, often coupled with psychotherapy, and return visits for boosters as needed.

Chronic Pain

As ketamine clinics pop up across the country, so do advertisements for ketamine for chronic pain relief. There is an abundance of research showing the benefit of ketamine for chronic pain (Orhurhu, Orhurhu, Bhatia, & Cohen, 2019), neuropathic pain (Hocking & Cousins, 2003; Pickering et al., 2020), and cancer pain (Culp, Kim, & Abdi, 2020).

Chronic pain is persistent pain where the ongoing pain causes significant life stress and includes ongoing headaches, lower back pain, arthritis, and neurogenic pain. A 2014 study points to the method of action as the inhibiting of the N-methyl-D-aspartate receptor (NMDA) (Niesters, Martini, & Dahan, 2014).

Research also supports the use of ketamine for acute pain, especially in emergency room setting as a stand-alone treatment or supplement to opioid treatment.

In 2018 the American Society of Anesthesiologists (Schaumburg, Illinois) along with the American Society of Regional Anesthesia and Pain Medicine (Pittsburgh, Pennsylvania), and the American Academy of Pain Medicine (Chicago, Illinois) issued guidelines for the use of intravenous ketamine for chronic pain (Cohen et al., 2018). While these guidelines provide useful training, approaches to patient monitoring, and general guidance on contraindications, they do not provide definitive guidance on dosing, patient selection, or a calculation of the risks of ongoing treatment. While generally safer than opioids, additional research continues to be needed.

Substance Use Disorders

Several studies have demonstrated promise for ketamine as a treatment for substance abuse disorder. Much of today's literature builds upon the 1997 study by Krupitsky and Grinenko from the Leningrad Regional Center for, Alcoholism and Drug Addiction

Therapy, which demonstrated that ketamine could promote abstinence in alcohol dependence and heroin dependence and reduce craving and self-administration of cocaine (Krupitsky & Grinenko, 1997).

In 2018, Ivan Ezquerra-Romano from University College London and his colleagues produced a study on ketamine for the treatment of addiction that was published in *Neuropharmacology* (Ivan Ezquerra-Romano, Lawn, Krupitsky, & Morgan, 2018). That same year, Jones et al from the Medical University of South Carolina published a systematic review of the efficacy of ketamine in the treatment of substance use disorders in *Front Psychiatry* (Jones, Mateus, Malcolm, Brady, & Back, 2018). This study showed that improvements were seen in all seven completed studies for alcohol use disorder, cocaine use disorder, and opioid use disorder.

Ravi Das, along with his colleagues, published a paper in *Nature Communications* in 2019 putting forth the notion that ketamine can reduce harmful drinking by pharmacologically rewriting drinking memories (Das et al., 2019). Drs. Worrell and Gould from Pennsylvania State University published a compelling 2021 paper on the therapeutic potential of ketamine for alcohol use disorder, analyzing 14 studies, and concluding that ketamine may be able to improve several of the neural changes seen with chronic alcohol use (Worrell & Gould, 2021).

Obsessive-Compulsive Disorder (OCD)

A 2020 study on ketamine for treatment-resistant obsessive-compulsive disorder suggested that ketamine could be a helpful treatment (Sharma et al., 2020). Out of 14 adult patients, one showed a dramatic positive response, two showed a moderately positive response, and 11 showed no clinical improvement. It's promising for people who do not respond to traditional OCD medication such as serotonin reuptake inhibitors, but more research is needed before ketamine becomes the go-to treatment.

Migraines

As ketamine clinics increase across the country, many are also advertising the treatment for migraines. There is some evidence that ketamine can treat migraines, but more research is needed on the topic (Bilhimer, Groth, & Holmes, 2020; Chah, Jones, Milord, Al-Eryani, & Enciso, 2021).

KETAMINE METHODS OF INTAKE

While most of the research on ketamine for depression uses infusions, the only FDA-approved method of intake is a nasal spray of esketamine. However, ketamine can also be taken orally, sublingually, and through intramuscular (IM) injections. While it's not suggested in a medical setting, recreational users sometimes snort ketamine. Below are the prominent methods of intake as supported by medical research.

IV (Infusions)

Most studies of ketamine for treatment-resistant depression use an IV drip, or infusion, as the method of intake. The administration of ketamine through an infusion is one of the most common methods of administration in medical settings. Infusions result in rapid uptake of the drug because it enters the bloodstream directly and bypasses the digestive system. In a 2019 study, patients with treatment-resistant depression received six infusions over the course of two weeks (Mandal, Sinha, & Goyal, 2019). There was significant improvement after the first dose, which continued through the month following treatment.

Many people receiving ketamine infusions are scheduled for six initial rounds and then come back for boosters as needed, ranging from every week to every two months. Usually given in a ketamine clinic or medical spa environment, the infusions can last anywhere from 40 minutes to an hour and a half. The dose is determined by weight and need, and the sessions are often coupled with psychotherapy and integration work.

Intramuscular Injection

Ketamine can be administered via intramuscular (IM) injection. Case reports from 2013 suggest that IM could offer the same quick and effective depression treatment as a ketamine IV treatment (Chilukuri et al., 2014). While more research is needed to support the efficacy of IM ketamine administration, it provides a welcome alternative for patients disinterested in or unable to use an IV line.

Intranasal

Currently, the only FDA-approved ketamine method of intake for treatment-resistant depression is a nasal spray of esketamine (Spravato). It can be self-administered by the patient under the supervision of a practitioner to ensure the patient's safety. Because ketamine and esketamine can have side effects such as dizziness and disorientation and has the potential for dependence, it's crucial that patients work closely with their providers while taking these medicines.

Ketamine consists of two molecular forms, R- and S-ketamine. Generically available ketamine is a mixture of both R- and S-ketamine. Esketamine consists only of the S- a form of ketamine, which research suggests has similar antidepressant effects to standard ketamine. Esketamine is a newer, patented medication that was studied and received FDA approval specifically for treatment-resistant depression.

Oral

Oral administration of ketamine is one of the most practical methods of intake, as it can be done at home and is available in generic form, so it is less expensive than the Spravato esketamine nasal spray. Tablets can be swallowed or placed under the tongue sublingually. This combination of increased convenience and reduced cost is leading to the popularity of this method, particularly for people with low to mid-levels of depression and anxiety. However, as reported in a 2019 paper, oral administration has its challenges with regard to dosing (Andrade, 2019). Because only 20%-30% of orally administered ketamine reaches the systemic circulation, it requires a larger dose than an infusion or injection.

WHAT RISKS ARE INVOLVED IN KETAMINE TREATMENTS?

The side effects of ketamine depend on several variables, including dosage and method of intake. As a result, it is important that you only use ketamine under the supervision of a qualified provider. Side effects of ketamine treatment include feeling out of body dizziness, altered perception, and euphoria. The most common side effect is nausea and vomiting.

It is difficult to overdose on ketamine, as demonstrated by its safety in anesthesia. As mobility may be impaired, do not drive after taking ketamine, and stay in a safe space while taking your medicine, ideally with a supervisor. Ketamine can be habit-forming, at least psychologically, as demonstrated by its use as a recreational drug, however, there is little evidence of this with clinical use.

Overuse of ketamine can result in bladder, urinary tract, and renal damage, which is why it's crucial to only use the medicine under the supervision of a trained clinician.

HOW MUCH DOES KETAMINE TREATMENT COST?

Cost is one of the biggest barriers to ketamine treatment. Insurers don't typically pay for it, and ketamine infusions can cost between $400 to $2,000 per treatment. Esketamine nasal spray can cost $590 and $885 per treatment session. As a result of this price, doctors will often work with a compound pharmacy to create an off-label ketamine nasal spray for patients at a lower price point.

Companies like HAPPŸŸ, Mindbloom, and nue.life have brought the cost down to closer to $200 per session by prescribing via telehealth and having the patients take their treatment at home.

KETAMINE-ASSISTED PSYCHOTHERAPY

When patients with treatment-resistant depression don't respond to traditional forms of therapy, they may turn to ketamine clinics for help. In addition to ketamine infusions, many clinics also offer integration work with a therapist or provide apps that digitally offer cognitive behavioral therapy, positive psychology, mindfulness, and other therapeutic guidance. However, because this is new and largely unregulated territory, the quality of services may vary widely. Some clinics may be staffed by qualified professionals who can provide high-quality care, while others may be less reputable and may not provide the same level of care. As a result, it's important for patients to do their research before choosing a clinic.

A 2018 study suggests that small doses of ketamine taken in-office with a therapist present can lower a person's inhibitions, allowing them to be more comfortable discussing trauma and accessing difficult emotions (Dore et al., 2019). The researchers acknowledge the benefits of both using ketamine in talk therapy with a provider present and in conjunction with out-of-office administration for treatment-resistant depression, PTSD, and other conditions.

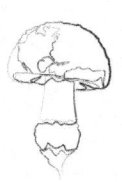

REFERENCES:

- Andrade, C. (2019). Oral Ketamine for Depression, 2. *The Journal of Clinical Psychiatry, 80*(2). doi:10.4088/jcp.19f12838
- Bilhimer, M. H., Groth, M. E., & Holmes, A. K. (2020). Ketamine for Migraine in the Emergency Department. *Adv Emerg Nurs J, 42*(2), 96-102. doi:10.1097/tme.0000000000000296
- Bystritsky, A. (2006). Treatment-resistant anxiety disorders. *Molecular Psychiatry, 11*(9), 805-814. doi:10.1038/sj.mp.4001852
- Chah, N., Jones, M., Milord, S., Al-Eryani, K., & Enciso, R. (2021). Efficacy of ketamine in the treatment of migraines and other unspecified primary headache disorders compared to placebo and other interventions: a systematic review. *J Dent Anesth Pain Med, 21*(5), 413-429. doi:10.17245/jdapm.2021.21.5.413
- Chilukuri, H., Reddy, N. P., Pathapati, R. M., Manu, A. N., Jollu, S., & Shaik, A. B. (2014). Acute antidepressant

effects of intramuscular versus intravenous ketamine. *Indian journal of psychological medicine, 36*(1), 71-76.
- Cohen, S. P., Bhatia, A., Buvanendran, A., Schwenk, E. S., Wasan, A. D., Hurley, R. W., . . . Hooten, W. M. (2018). Consensus Guidelines on the Use of Intravenous Ketamine Infusions for Chronic Pain From the American Society of Regional Anesthesia and Pain Medicine, the American Academy of Pain Medicine, and the American Society of Anesthesiologists. *Reg Anesth Pain Med, 43*(5), 521-546. doi:10.1097/aap.0000000000000808
- Culp, C., Kim, H. K., & Abdi, S. (2020). Ketamine Use for Cancer and Chronic Pain Management. *Frontiers in pharmacology, 11*, 599721. doi:10.3389/fphar.2020.599721
- D'Anci, K. E., Uhl, S., Giradi, G., & Martin, C. (2019). Treatments for the Prevention and Management of Suicide: A Systematic Review. *Ann Intern Med, 171*(5), 334-342. doi:10.7326/m19-0869
- Das, R. K., Gale, G., Walsh, K., Hennessy, V. E., Iskandar, G., Mordecai, L. A., . . . Kamboj, S. K. (2019). Ketamine can reduce harmful drinking by pharmacologically rewriting drinking memories. *Nature Communications, 10*(1), 5187. doi:10.1038/s41467-019-13162-w
- Domany, Y., Bleich-Cohen, M., Tarrasch, R., Meidan, R., Litvak-Lazar, O., Stoppleman, N., . . . Sharon, H. (2018). Repeated oral ketamine for out-patient treatment of resistant depression: randomised, double-blind, placebo-controlled, proof-of-concept study. *The British Journal of Psychiatry, 214*, 1-7. doi:10.1192/bjp.2018.196
- Dore, J., Turnipseed, B., Dwyer, S., Turnipseed, A., Andries, J., Ascani, G., . . . Wolfson, P. (2019). Ketamine Assisted Psychotherapy (KAP): Patient Demographics, Clinical Data and Outcomes in Three Large Practices Administering Ketamine with Psychotherapy. *Journal of*

- *Psychoactive Drugs, 51*(2), 189-198. doi:10.1080/02791072.2019.1587556
- Feder, A., Costi, S., Rutter, S. B., Collins, A. B., Govindarajulu, U., Jha, M. K., . . . Charney, D. S. (2021). A Randomized Controlled Trial of Repeated Ketamine Administration for Chronic Posttraumatic Stress Disorder. *Am J Psychiatry, 178*(2), 193-202. doi:10.1176/appi.ajp.2020.20050596
- Garakani, A., Murrough, J. W., Freire, R. C., Thom, R. P., Larkin, K., Buono, F. D., & Iosifescu, D. V. (2020). Pharmacotherapy of Anxiety Disorders: Current and Emerging Treatment Options. *Front Psychiatry, 11*, 595584. doi:10.3389/fpsyt.2020.595584
- Glue, P., Medlicott, N. J., Neehoff, S., Surman, P., Lam, F., Hung, N., & Hung, C.-T. (2020). Safety and efficacy of extended release ketamine tablets in patients with treatment-resistant depression and anxiety: open label pilot study. *Therapeutic Advances in Psychopharmacology, 10*, 2045125320922474. doi:10.1177/2045125320922474
- Hocking, G., & Cousins, M. J. (2003). Ketamine in Chronic Pain Management: An Evidence-Based Review. *Anesthesia & Analgesia, 97*(6). Retrieved from https://journals.lww.com/anesthesia-analgesia/Fulltext/2003/12000/Ketamine_in_Chronic_Pain_Management__An.37.aspx
- Irwin, S. A., Iglewicz, A., Nelesen, R. A., Lo, J. Y., Carr, C. H., Romero, S. D., & Lloyd, L. S. (2013). Daily Oral Ketamine for the Treatment of Depression and Anxiety in Patients Receiving Hospice Care: A 28-Day Open-Label Proof-of-Concept Trial. *Journal of Palliative Medicine, 16*(8), 958-965. doi:10.1089/jpm.2012.0617
- Ivan Ezquerra-Romano, I., Lawn, W., Krupitsky, E., & Morgan, C. J. A. (2018). Ketamine for the treatment of addiction: Evidence and potential mechanisms.

Neuropharmacology, 142, 72-82. doi:10.1016/j.neuropharm.2018.01.017

- Jones, J. L., Mateus, C. F., Malcolm, R. J., Brady, K. T., & Back, S. E. (2018). Efficacy of Ketamine in the Treatment of Substance Use Disorders: A Systematic Review. *Front Psychiatry, 9*, 277. doi:10.3389/fpsyt.2018.00277
- Krupitsky, E. M., & Grinenko, A. Y. (1997). Ketamine Psychedelic Therapy (KPT): A Review of the Results of Ten Years of Research. *Journal of Psychoactive Drugs, 29*(2), 165-183. doi:10.1080/02791072.1997.10400185
- Mandal, S., Sinha, V. K., & Goyal, N. (2019). Efficacy of ketamine therapy in the treatment of depression. *Indian journal of psychiatry, 61*(5), 480-485. doi:10.4103/psychiatry.IndianJPsychiatry_484_18
- Niesters, M., Martini, C., & Dahan, A. (2014). Ketamine for chronic pain: risks and benefits. *British journal of clinical pharmacology, 77*(2), 357-367. doi:10.1111/bcp.12094
- Orhurhu, V., Orhurhu, M. S., Bhatia, A., & Cohen, S. P. (2019). Ketamine Infusions for Chronic Pain: A Systematic Review and Meta-analysis of Randomized Controlled Trials. *Anesth Analg, 129*(1), 241-254. doi:10.1213/ane.0000000000004185
- Pickering, G., Pereira, B., Morel, V., Corriger, A., Giron, F., Marcaillou, F., . . . Delage, N. (2020). Ketamine and Magnesium for Refractory Neuropathic Pain: A Randomized, Double-blind, Crossover Trial. *Anesthesiology, 133*(1), 154-164. doi:10.1097/aln.0000000000003345
- Sharma, L. P., Thamby, A., Balachander, S., Janardhanan, C. N., Jaisoorya, T. S., Arumugham, S. S., & Reddy, Y. C. J. (2020). Clinical utility of repeated intravenous ketamine treatment for resistant obsessive-compulsive disorder. *Asian J Psychiatr, 52*, 102183. doi:10.1016/j.ajp.2020.102183

- Worrell, S. D., & Gould, T. J. (2021). Therapeutic potential of ketamine for alcohol use disorder. *Neurosci Biobehav Rev, 126*, 573-589. doi:10.1016/j.neubiorev.2021.05.006
- Zanos, P., & Gould, T. D. (2018). Mechanisms of ketamine action as an antidepressant. *Mol Psychiatry, 23*(4), 801-811. doi:10.1038/mp.2017.255

SIXTEEN
AT-HOME, SUBLINGUAL KETAMINE STUDY RESULTS
MATT ZEMON, MSC

MEDICALLY REVIEWED BY DR. DAVID FLYNN, MD, MBA, CPHQ

In July 2022, as this book was in its final preparations for publication, a study of 1,247 participants using at-home, sublingual ketamine was published in the peer-reviewed Journal of Affective Disorders (Hull et al., 2022). Participants all received ketamine-assisted therapy at home over a four-week period. This study, the largest of its kind to date on the real-world safety and effectiveness of at-home sublingual ketamine-assisted therapy, demonstrated promising results, including the following highlights:

- 89% of the participants experienced an improvement in symptoms of depression and anxiety.
- 63% of participants showed a reduction in symptoms of 50% or more.
- Nearly 80% of patients who reported suicidal ideation at baseline no longer reported any suicidal ideation after four sessions.
- Less than 5% of participants reported side effects.

Before proceeding, it is important to be aware that while the results in this study are promising and this study was published in a peer-reviewed journal, four of the ten authors were employees of the service providing the data, two received minor consulting fees from the service provider, and two are on the service provider's scientific advisory board. Matteo Malgaroli, PhD from the Department of Psychiatry at NYU Grossman's School of Medicine, and Adam Gazzaley, MD, PhD, distinguished professor of Neurology, Physiology, and Psychiatry from the University of California, had no competing interests. This chapter summarizes the results and importance of this recent study for people considering utilizing an at-home ketamine provider.

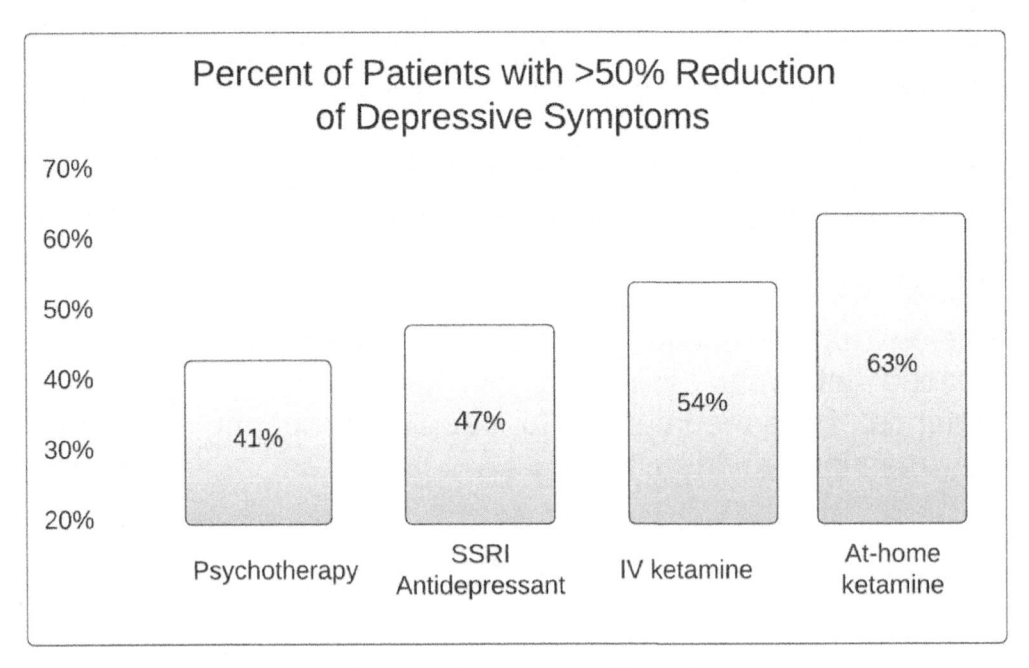

Percent of Patients with >50% Reduction of Depressive Symptoms

Treatment	Percent
Psychotherapy	41%
SSRI Antidepressant	47%
IV ketamine	54%
At-home ketamine	63%

*At-home ketamine was 34% more effective than SSRI antidepressants

*At-home ketamine was 54% more effective than psychotherapy

*At-home ketamine was 17% more effective than IV ketamine, despite lower cost and non-clinical setting

*At-home ketamine results reported after 4 weeks. SSRI and psychotherapy required 2+ months to achieve reported results.

BACKGROUND

Over 33% of people suffer from some anxiety, and it is well documented that anxiety plays a role in depression, physical illness, and substance abuse (Bandelow & Michaelis, 2015). Existing treatments, both pharmacological and non-pharmacological, are not effective for almost 40% of the population (Bystritsky, 2006), and the pharmacological options take up to 14 weeks for onset of action (Gorman & Kent, 1999). While selective serotonin reuptake inhibitors (SSRIs) are the most commonly prescribed anti-anxiety medications (Ansara, 2020), researchers have been studying the use of subanesthetic doses of ketamine, an N-methyl-D-aspartate (NMDA) receptor antagonist, as an alternative (Grady, Marsh, Tenhouse, & Klein, 2018).

Ketamine is lipid and water-soluble, allowing it to be administered in a variety of modes, including intravenous (IV), intramuscular injection (IM), intranasally, and by mouth, rectal, subcutaneous, and epidural routes (Craven, 2007). Ketamine has a relatively short therapeutic effect, typically lasting 1-2 weeks and therefore requiring repeated dosing (Corriger & Pickering, 2019). IV and IM administration have superior bioavailability and dose control but require trained professionals to administer, adding expense and inconvenience (Gao, Rejaei, & Liu, 2016).

Oral, sublingual at-home ketamine therapy offers a promising, needle-free alternative to expensive IV and IM ketamine and a potential alternative to SSRIs and other existing pharmacological interventions for treating depression and anxiety. This method of administration has been used for years with chronic pain management (Peltoniemi, Hagelberg, Olkkola, & Saari, 2016) and has a low risk of abuse (Farré & Camí, 1991). When equivalently dosed, studies have not found meaningful differences in efficacy based on routes of administration (Chilukuri et al., 2014; Romeo, Choucha, Fossati, & Rotge, 2015).

As little as one-tenth of a general anesthetic dose of ketamine can create psychedelic experiences with the perception of floating, disconnection from surroundings, becoming separated from the body, and going to a different world (Collier, 1972). While some researchers believe this dissociative effect is necessary for its antidepressant effects, the current research is divided (Cooper et al., 2017). Classic psychedelics can cause similar effects as ketamine, however, ketamine is the only psychedelic that is currently legal to prescribe for anxiety and depression, albeit off-label (Dore et al., 2019).

Given the number of people impacted by depression and anxiety disorders and the high rates of the inefficacy of existing therapeutic options, new treatments are needed. Oral ketamine, which is affordable and can be self-administered, is being promoted as an alternative, but until recently, there have been no large studies supporting its safety and efficacy. As summarized in Table 1, prior to this study, multiple studies demonstrated promising results regarding the effectiveness of oral ketamine for depression and anxiety symptoms but had small sample sizes, various dosages and administration frequencies, and inconsistent results. This study, with its large sample size and more consistent dosing and administration, reported significantly more consistent results.

PRESCRIBING IN STUDY

Patients met virtually with a prescribing clinician who held current prescribing privileges in their state(s) or licensure and had demonstrated psychiatric training. Clinicians included psychiatrists, psychiatric-mental health nurse practitioners, and physician assistants with psychiatry experience. The prescribing clinician was responsible for determining whether the patient was suitable for at-home ketamine treatment based on answers to an online screening questionnaire and the standard medical and psychiatric evaluation that took place through a live video conference.

STUDY PARTICIPATION

The study participants were adults between the ages of 19 and 76 whose primary complaint was anxiety and/or depression. Study participants were recruited primarily from digital advertisements and paid to participate in this program. The mean average age was 40; women comprised 54.6% of the participants. Based on the video interview and assessment scores, participants received a depression or anxiety diagnosis from their licensed clinician.

There were a number of reasons participants were not accepted into this treatment program, including:

1. Allergies to ketamine.
2. Alcohol or substance use dependence.
3. History of opioid use disorder.
4. Active psychotic, manic, or mixed symptoms or history of psychotic symptoms.
5. Untreated high blood pressure.
6. Congestive heart failure or other serious cardiac problems.
7. Severe breathing problems.
8. Unstable thyroid disease.
9. Elevated intraocular pressure/glaucoma.
10. Elevated intracranial pressure.
11. Other serious medical illnesses.
12. Pregnancy, nursing, or currently trying to become pregnant.
13. Active suicidal ideation with the method, intent, or plan within the past month or a suicide attempt within the past year.
14. Any other aspect of the patient's psychiatric history, outpatient support system, or home environment that would render at-home treatment psychologically unsafe in the opinion of the prescribing clinician, including a history of severe and unresolved trauma.

GUIDES

Guides were not licensed therapists but were required to have prior behavioral coaching experience and relevant certifications. In addition to the experience the guides brought, these non-medical facilitators were trained in patient support by the telehealth provider.

KETAMINE THERAPY PROCESS

Prescribing clinicians and patients met for 40-60 minutes to determine whether the patient qualified for the at-home program. Those that were accepted were sent an initial dose of sublingual, rapid dissolving ketamine to establish a baseline dosing along with ondansetron for potential nausea. The initial dosing was based on the IV ketamine standard of 0.5 mg/kg, which was then adjusted up to account for the lower (20%) bioavailability of sublingual ketamine.

After the initial dose, dosing was adjusted up to 5 mg/kg to achieve the desired dissociative goal, similar to what was seen with intravenous (IV) and intramuscular (IM) treatments, with the hypothesis that greater levels of dissociation predict stronger and longer lasting antidepressant effects.

Participants prepared for this treatment with a 30-minute video call with their guide, reinforcing the education provided by the prescribing clinician and helping to establish the patient's mindset ("Set") for the medication session. During the initial meeting, patients confirmed a peer monitor's presence for their session. They typically used a trusted friend or family member. The guide also provided training to the peer monitor on how to best support the patient.

Patients confirmed they had blood pressure under 150/100 and a heart rate under 100 using a home blood pressure monitor. They were asked to fast for at least three hours before their medication session and to refrain from liquids for at least one hour. Alcohol, stimulants, and benzodiazepines were to be avoided on the day of treatment.

For this study, patients were asked to hold the medication under their tongue or between their cheeks and gums for seven minutes without swallowing. After seven minutes, they were instructed to spit out all the saliva that had formed. This approach greatly reduces the amount of medication swallowed by the patient. Swallowing can increase the ketamine metabolites in the body, leading to prolonged sedation and increased nausea. There was no monitoring of the patients' adherence to the seven minutes, and this amount of time is lower than the 12-15 minutes used by other large practitioners (Dore et al., 2019) and recommended by the Ketamine Training Center.

After spitting out the saliva, patients laid down, put on an eye mask, and listened to music for approximately one hour. After their initial session, they journaled and then met again with their guide for 20 to 30 minutes to integrate their experience.

A second meeting with their clinician took place one to two days later and a second integration session with their guide.

Following these meetings, the patients communicated with their guides via text and were able to request additional clinician meetings as needed.

COST PER SESSION

The cost for these at-home sessions ranged from $193 to $250 per treatment, which is reported as 28% to 83% of the price of a single ketamine infusion in a clinic.

ASSESSMENTS USED IN STUDY

Participants took the 9-item Patient Health Questionnaire (PHQ-9) for depression (Kroenke, Spitzer, Williams, Monahan, & Löwe, 2007) and the 7-item Generalized Disorder questionnaire (GAD-7) for anxiety (Spitzer, Kroenke, Williams, & Löwe, 2006). The 5-item Columbia Suicide Severity Rating Scale (C-SSRS) was used for measuring suicidal ideation (Kelly Posner et al., 2011). Alcohol use was assessed using AUDIT, the 10-item Alcohol Use Disorders Identification Test (Bush et al.) and substance use was assessed by the DAST-10, the 10-item Drug Abuse Screening Test (Villalobos-Gallegos, Pérez-López, Mendoza-Hassey, Graue-Moreno, & Marín-Navarrete, 2015). Side effects and adverse events were assessed through a single-item self-report questionnaire administered twice. Dissociative symptoms were measured with three items adapted from the Clinician-Administered Dissociative States Scale (CADSS), focusing on how disconnected physically and mentally the patient felt (Bremner et al., 1998).

Baseline PHQ-9 scores showed that participants were predominately in the moderate-severe category for depression, while baseline CAD-9 scores indicated that most participants were in the severe category for anxiety.

SIDE EFFECTS AND ADVERSE EVENTS

Side effects, tolerability, and abuse potential play a role in oral ketamine's overall effectiveness and safety. Out of the 1,247 patients included in the study, 59 reported side effects after session two (4.7%) and 27 after session four (3.8%). Four patients had their treatment discontinued due to adverse events, and two were removed from treatment due to non-compliance.

Ketamine has been used as a street drug since the 1960s, and in both human and animal studies, it has been demonstrated that there is potential for misuse (Liu, Lin, Wu, & Zhou, 2016). Due to its rapid and intense effects, misuse potential is higher with inhalation than with oral administration, but oral administration does not eliminate this risk (Argoff, Stanos, & Wieman, 2013). There is also increased potential for addiction and tolerance for patients that need multiple treatments of ketamine to maintain its efficacy (Schak et al., 2016). The abuse potential may be increased for at-home administration of ketamine, though there was no evidence of misuse in this study.

OBSERVATIONS

The results for at-home sublingual ketamine are similar to studies for IV ketamine (Lee, Della Selva, Liu, & Himelhoch, 2015; McInnes, Qian, Gargeya, DeBattista, & Heifets, 2022). Response and remission rates range from similar to stronger than in previous studies (aan het Rot et al., 2010; Fava et al., 2020; Lener, Kadriu, & Zarate, 2017; McInnes et al., 2022; Phillips et al., 2019). This is understandable as multiple studies show that individuals with lower baseline scores are more likely to achieve the criteria for response and remission. Results being stronger than lab studies is likely related to the repeated administration versus the single dose typically administered in a lab.

While women outnumber men 2-to-1 for antidepressant use and 4-to-1 for psychological treatments (Brody & Gu, 2020), 45% of the participants in this study were men, further suggesting that men are more likely to use medication-based treatments over psychosocial programs. Based on this, this approach may reach a portion of the population that has been undertreated for anxiety and depression.

Participants in this study demonstrated rapid and consistent effects, which is significantly different from the results found in monoaminergic treatments, which can produce similar remission rates in up to 10 to 14 weeks but have highly variable rates of effectiveness (Fournier et al., 2010). Psychotherapies take 12 to 16 weeks to achieve a slightly weaker rate of change than reported here (Kryst et al., 2020).

Researchers are divided as to whether dissociative experiences help or hinder the effectiveness of ketamine as a mental health treatment (Cooper et al., 2017; Niciu et al., 2018). This study showed evidence that greater dissociative experiences at the end of treatment decreased the likelihood of symptom improvement. This is in line with Valentine's research (Valentine et al., 2011) but different from Luckenbaugh's findings which suggested that only the dissociative effects predicted a more robust and sustained antidepressant effect (Luckenbaugh et al., 2014).

CONCLUSION

Given the number of people impacted by depression and anxiety disorders and the high rates of the inefficacy of existing therapeutic options, new treatments are needed. Oral ketamine, which is affordable and can be self-administered, appears promising but has historically lacked quality supporting data. Despite the limitations of the study design, this study provides evidence that at-home ketamine is safe, fast, and effective for most patients. This research should be seen as another step in building evidence around the effectiveness, safety, and tolerability of at-home oral ketamine for the symptoms of depression and anxiety, and further investigations using randomized controlled trials are necessary to establish further the comparative effectiveness and safety against the current pharmacological and non-pharmacological therapeutic options.

Table 1: Studies on the efficacy of oral ketamine for symptoms of anxiety

Clinical population	Author	Study design	Primary focus	N	Ketamine type & dose	Outcome measures	Time Period	Results
Palliative Care	Irwin et al. (2010)	Case series	Anxiety symptoms	2	One dose of .5 mg/kg oral ketamine	HADS, HRSD	15 days	Anxiety symptoms improved within 1 hours and sustained for up to 1 week
Palliative Care	Irwin et al. (2013)	Open-label, proof-of-concept	Anxiety symptoms	14	Daily doses of .5/mg/kg oral ketamine in cherry syrup	HADS	28 days	By day 3 there were significant reductions in anxiety symptoms in 100% of completers. Mean TTR was 8.6 days. Maintained well through end-of-study.
Palliative Care	McNulty & Hahn (2012)	Case Report	Severe constant anxiety	1	Single-dose of .5 mg/kg subcutaneous followed by 40 mg/5 mL oral ketamine daily.	Self Self-reported rating between 1 and 10	11 weeks	Full anxiety and depression relief within 1 hour of injection. Oral started on day 4. Depression still at 0 and anxiety is labile.
Palliative Care	Swiatek et al. (2016)	Case Report	Anxiety	1	.25 mg/kg (5 mg total every 8 hours)	HADS-D	14 days	38% improvement that deteriorated along with patient physical health. Family chose to not continue after 9 days.
Palliative Care	Iglewicz et al. (2015)	Retrospective review	Global improvement	31	22 patients received a single dose of .5 mg/kg and five received two doses. Three received 3x/day each day studied.	CGI	21 days	93% positive results within 3 days, 60% in days 8-21

Referred TRD patients	Al Shirawi et al. (2017)	Retrospective review	Treatment-resistant MDD	22	50 mg titrated upward by 25 mg at each dose (every 3 days)	BDI-II	28 days	Modest effectiveness. 45% showed up to a 20% negative reduction in mood.
Out-patients referred by community or hospital	Domany et al. (2018)	Double-blind, randomized, placebo-controlled trial	Major depressive disorder	41	1 mg/kg non-flavoured oral ketamine 3x/week	MADRS	28 days	Reduction of 12.75 points. 23.75% of the ketamine group went into remission. No patients in control went into remission.
Trial Group	Glue et al. (2020)	Open-label pilot study	Major depressive disorder and/or social anxiety disorder	7	Extended-release oral ketamine between 60 mg and 240 mg based on individual response	HAMA and MADRS	3 days	100% showed a reduction in HAMA or MADRS of 50% or greater. 6 out of 7 had reduction greater than 50% in fear response
Referred TRD patients	Hartberg et al. (2018)	Retrospective review	Major depressive disorder and/or	37	Sublingual dose of .5 mg/kg the doses of .5 mg/kg-7.0 mg/kg mixed with a flavoured drink	K10	3 years	65% reduction in new admissions and 70% reduction in hospital stays
Private practice	Dore et al. (2019)	Retrospective review	Moderate anxiety	235	SL ketamine as troche or a rapid-dissolve tablet (average 200-250 mg), sometimes following initial IM session (80-90 mg). Some patients had IM sessions intermixed.	HAMA, BDI	5 years	Average reduction of 5.5 points on HAMA from moderate to mild

Notes: BDI, Beck Depression Inventory; BDI-II, Beck Depression Inventory II; CGI, Clinical Global Impressions Scale; HADS, Hospital Anxiety and Depression Scale; HADS-D, Hospital Anxiety and Depression Scale subscale for depression; HAMA, Hamilton Anxiety Rating Scale; HRSD, Hamilton Rating Scale for Depression; K10, Kessler Psychological Distress Scale, MADRS. Montgomery-Asberg Depression Rating Scale;

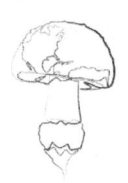

REFERENCES:

- aan het Rot, M., Collins, K. A., Murrough, J. W., Perez, A. M., Reich, D. L., Charney, D. S., & Mathew, S. J. (2010). Safety and efficacy of repeated-dose intravenous ketamine for treatment-resistant depression. *Biol Psychiatry, 67*(2), 139-145. doi:10.1016/j.biopsych.2009.08.038
- Ansara, E. D. (2020). Management of treatment-resistant generalized anxiety disorder. *The mental health clinician, 10*(6), 326-334. doi:10.9740/mhc.2020.11.326
- Argoff, C. E., Stanos, S. P., & Wieman, M. S. (2013). Validity testing of patient objections to acceptance of tamper-resistant opioid formulations. *J Pain Res, 6*, 367-373. doi:10.2147/jpr.S37343
- Bandelow, B., & Michaelis, S. (2015). Epidemiology of anxiety disorders in the 21st century. *Dialogues in clinical neuroscience, 17*(3), 327-335. doi:10.31887/DCNS.2015.17.3/bbandelow
- Bremner, J. D., Krystal, J. H., Putnam, F. W., Southwick, S. M., Marmar, C., Charney, D. S., & Mazure, C. M. (1998). Measurement of dissociative states with the clinician-administered dissociative states scale (CADSS). *Journal of Traumatic Stress: Official Publication of The International Society for Traumatic Stress Studies, 11*(1), 125-136.
- Brody, D. J., & Gu, Q. (2020). *Antidepressant use among adults: United States, 2015-2018*: US Department of Health and Human Services, Centers for Disease Control and ....

- Bush, K., Kivlahan, D., McDonell, M., Fihn, S., Bradley, K., & Project, A. C. Q. I. AUDIT alcohol consumption questions (AUDITC): An effective brief screening test for problem drinking. Alcohol Use Disorders Identification Test. *Arch Intern Med.*
- Bystritsky, A. (2006). Treatment-resistant anxiety disorders. *Molecular Psychiatry, 11*(9), 805-814. doi:10.1038/sj.mp.4001852
- Chilukuri, H., Reddy, N. P., Pathapati, R. M., Manu, A. N., Jollu, S., & Shaik, A. B. (2014). Acute antidepressant effects of intramuscular versus intravenous ketamine. *Indian journal of psychological medicine, 36*(1), 71-76.
- Collier, B. B. (1972). Ketamine and the conscious mind. *Anaesthesia, 27*(2), 120-134. doi:10.1111/j.1365-2044.1972.tb08186.x
- Cooper, M. D., Rosenblat, J. D., Cha, D. S., Lee, Y., Kakar, R., & McIntyre, R. S. (2017). Strategies to mitigate dissociative and psychotomimetic effects of ketamine in the treatment of major depressive episodes: a narrative review. *The World Journal of Biological Psychiatry, 18*(6), 410-423.
- Corriger, A., & Pickering, G. (2019). Ketamine and depression: a narrative review. *Drug Des Devel Ther, 13*, 3051-3067. doi:10.2147/dddt.S221437
- Craven, R. (2007). Ketamine. *Anaesthesia, 62 Suppl 1*, 48-53. doi:10.1111/j.1365-2044.2007.05298.x
- Dore, J., Turnipseed, B., Dwyer, S., Turnipseed, A., Andries, J., Ascani, G., . . . Wolfson, P. (2019). Ketamine Assisted Psychotherapy (KAP): Patient Demographics, Clinical Data and Outcomes in Three Large Practices Administering Ketamine with Psychotherapy. *Journal of Psychoactive Drugs, 51*(2), 189-198. doi:10.1080/02791072.2019.1587556
- Farré, M., & Camí, J. (1991). Pharmacokinetic considerations in abuse liability evaluation. *Br J Addict,*

- *86*(12), 1601-1606. doi:10.1111/j.1360-0443.1991.tb01754.x
- Fava, M., Freeman, M. P., Flynn, M., Judge, H., Hoeppner, B. B., Cusin, C., . . . Iosifescu, D. V. (2020). Double-blind, placebo-controlled, dose-ranging trial of intravenous ketamine as adjunctive therapy in treatment-resistant depression (TRD). *Molecular Psychiatry, 25*(7), 1592-1603.
- Fournier, J. C., DeRubeis, R. J., Hollon, S. D., Dimidjian, S., Amsterdam, J. D., Shelton, R. C., & Fawcett, J. (2010). Antidepressant drug effects and depression severity: a patient-level meta-analysis. *Jama, 303*(1), 47-53.
- Gao, M., Rejaei, D., & Liu, H. (2016). Ketamine use in current clinical practice. *Acta pharmacologica Sinica, 37*(7), 865-872. doi:10.1038/aps.2016.5
- Gorman, J. M., & Kent, J. M. (1999). SSRIs and SNRIs: broad spectrum of efficacy beyond major depression. *J Clin Psychiatry, 60 Suppl 4*, 33-38; discussion 39.
- Grady, S. E., Marsh, T. A., Tenhouse, A., & Klein, K. (2018). Ketamine for the treatment of major depressive disorder and bipolar depression: A review of the literature. *The mental health clinician, 7*(1), 16-23. doi:10.9740/mhc.2017.01.016
- Hull, T. D., Malgaroli, M., Gazzaley, A., Akiki, T. J., Madan, A., Vando, L., . . . Paleos, C. (2022). At-home, sublingual ketamine telehealth is a safe and effective treatment for moderate to severe anxiety and depression: Findings from a large, prospective, open-label effectiveness trial. *J Affect Disord, 314*, 59-67. doi:10.1016/j.jad.2022.07.004
- Kelly Posner, Ph.D. ,, Gregory K. Brown, Ph.D. ,, Barbara Stanley, Ph.D. ,, David A. Brent, M.D. ,, Kseniya V. Yershova, Ph.D. ,, Maria A. Oquendo, M.D. ,, . . . J. John Mann, M.D. (2011). The Columbia–Suicide Severity Rating Scale: Initial Validity and Internal Consistency Findings From Three Multisite Studies With Adolescents and Adults.

American Journal of Psychiatry, 168(12), 1266-1277. doi:10.1176/appi.ajp.2011.10111704

- Kroenke, K., Spitzer, R. L., Williams, J. B. W., Monahan, P. O., & Löwe, B. (2007). Anxiety Disorders in Primary Care: Prevalence, Impairment, Comorbidity, and Detection. *Annals of Internal Medicine, 146*(5), 317-325. doi:10.7326/0003-4819-146-5-200703060-00004

- Kryst, J., Kawalec, P., Mitoraj, A. M., Pilc, A., Lasoń, W., & Brzostek, T. (2020). Efficacy of single and repeated administration of ketamine in unipolar and bipolar depression: a meta-analysis of randomized clinical trials. *Pharmacological Reports, 72*(3), 543-562.

- Lee, E. E., Della Selva, M. P., Liu, A., & Himelhoch, S. (2015). Ketamine as a novel treatment for major depressive disorder and bipolar depression: a systematic review and quantitative meta-analysis. *General hospital psychiatry, 37*(2), 178-184.

- Lener, M. S., Kadriu, B., & Zarate, C. A. (2017). Ketamine and beyond: investigations into the potential of glutamatergic agents to treat depression. *Drugs, 77*(4), 381-401.

- Liu, Y., Lin, D., Wu, B., & Zhou, W. (2016). Ketamine abuse potential and use disorder. *Brain Res Bull, 126*(Pt 1), 68-73. doi:10.1016/j.brainresbull.2016.05.016

- Luckenbaugh, D. A., Niciu, M. J., Ionescu, D. F., Nolan, N. M., Richards, E. M., Brutsche, N. E., . . . Zarate, C. A. (2014). Do the dissociative side effects of ketamine mediate its antidepressant effects? *Journal of Affective Disorders, 159*, 56-61.

- McInnes, L. A., Qian, J. J., Gargeya, R. S., DeBattista, C., & Heifets, B. D. (2022). A retrospective analysis of ketamine intravenous therapy for depression in real-world care settings. *Journal of Affective Disorders, 301*, 486-495.

- Niciu, M. J., Shovestul, B. J., Jaso, B. A., Farmer, C., Luckenbaugh, D. A., Brutsche, N. E., . . . Zarate Jr, C. A. (2018). Features of dissociation differentially predict antidepressant response to ketamine in treatment-resistant depression. *Journal of Affective Disorders, 232*, 310-315.
- Peltoniemi, M. A., Hagelberg, N. M., Olkkola, K. T., & Saari, T. I. (2016). Ketamine: A Review of Clinical Pharmacokinetics and Pharmacodynamics in Anesthesia and Pain Therapy. *Clin Pharmacokinet, 55*(9), 1059-1077. doi:10.1007/s40262-016-0383-6
- Phillips, J. L., Norris, S., Talbot, J., Birmingham, M., Hatchard, T., Ortiz, A., . . . Blier, P. (2019). Single, repeated, and maintenance ketamine infusions for treatment-resistant depression: a randomized controlled trial. *American Journal of Psychiatry, 176*(5), 401-409.
- Romeo, B., Choucha, W., Fossati, P., & Rotge, J.-Y. (2015). Meta-analysis of short-and mid-term efficacy of ketamine in unipolar and bipolar depression. *Psychiatry research, 230*(2), 682-688.
- Schak, K. M., Vande Voort, J. L., Johnson, E. K., Kung, S., Leung, J. G., Rasmussen, K. G., . . . Frye, M. A. (2016). Potential Risks of Poorly Monitored Ketamine Use in Depression Treatment. *American Journal of Psychiatry, 173*(3), 215-218. doi:10.1176/appi.ajp.2015.15081082
- Spitzer, R. L., Kroenke, K., Williams, J. B. W., & Löwe, B. (2006). A Brief Measure for Assessing Generalized Anxiety Disorder: The GAD-7. *Archives of Internal Medicine, 166*(10), 1092-1097. doi:10.1001/archinte.166.10.1092
- Valentine, G. W., Mason, G. F., Gomez, R., Fasula, M., Watzl, J., Pittman, B., . . . Sanacora, G. (2011). The antidepressant effect of ketamine is not associated with changes in occipital amino acid neurotransmitter content as measured by [1H]-MRS. *Psychiatry Research: Neuroimaging, 191*(2), 122-127.

- Villalobos-Gallegos, L., Pérez-López, A., Mendoza-Hassey, R., Graue-Moreno, J., & Marín-Navarrete, R. (2015). Psychometric and diagnostic properties of the Drug Abuse Screening Test (DAST): Comparing the DAST-20 vs. the DAST-10. *Salud mental, 38*(2), 89-94.

SEVENTEEN
KETAMINE AND TREATMENT-RESISTANT DEPRESSION
AMELIA WALSH

MEDICALLY REVIEWED BY DR. DAVID FLYNN, MD, MBA, CPHQ

Ketamine is a medication that has been used for decades as an anesthetic, but it has also shown promise as a treatment for depression. Depression is the most common cause of disability, but many people do not find adequate relief from conventional treatments. In recent years, interest in ketamine has grown alongside evidence that it can provide rapid relief to people with treatment-resistant depression. While traditional antidepressants can take weeks or months to take effect, ketamine works quickly, often providing relief within hours. Additionally, ketamine has a low risk of side effects and appears to be effective even in people who have not responded to other treatments. As a result, ketamine represents a potentially transformative treatment for depression, and the innovation of its use for treating different forms of depression has become increasingly more interesting as it is evident that it can provide rapid relief to persons with treatment-resistant depression.

Depression is the cause of disability, but many people experience side effects or do not find adequate relief from conventional treatments. It is estimated that 10-30% are resistant to the beneficial effects of traditional antidepressants

Here are answers to some of the most common questions about the possibility of adding ketamine to a course of treatment for depression.

HOW DOES KETAMINE WORK FOR DEPRESSION?

Ketamine is an exciting development because it acts rapidly and tends to produce robust beneficial effects when it does work. Most antidepressants can take weeks to achieve full results, and their overall effects are often modest. The opportunity to quickly achieve a significant improvement is a welcome innovation.

Ketamine may help repair connections in the brain by inducing a state of neuron plasticity, allowing the potential for significant shifts in negative mood states as well as longer-term change.

Ketamine is not a lifetime commitment when it works well; it is a series of treatments that occur over a relatively short period of time (depending on the case) and can offer lasting symptom relief if successful.

Ketamine for bipolar depression

Bipolar depression is one of the most likely psychiatric conditions to cause suicidal ideation and be resistant to treatment. Ketamine has been studied with mood stabilizers such as lithium or valproic acid and is shown to be effective for bipolar depression (Wilkowska, Szałach, & Cubała, 2020). It has some promising studies showing rapid anti-suicidal effects. Use for serious mood disorders such as those with suicidality should be attempted only under the supervision of professionals with close monitoring.

Ketamine for severe and treatment-resistant depression

Typical antidepressants work on what is called the monoamine system, targeting neurotransmitters like dopamine, norepinephrine, and serotonin (Ansara, 2020). They are typically a successful form of treatment for depression, but those suffering from major depressive disorder (MDD) can sometimes be resistant to treatment and be candidates for additional methods of therapy.

Ketamine can be effective for major and clinical cases of depression when traditional methods have failed (Serafini, Howland, Rovedi, Girardi, & Amore, 2014). It can also be used safely and effectively in conjunction with traditional antidepressants; in fact, this is how the FDA-approved ketamine nasal inhaler, esketamine (Spravato) is intended to be used (FDA, 2019). In cases of severe depression, ketamine has offered rapid relief of symptoms in controlled medical studies with transient or short-lived side effects around the time of ketamine administration (Short, Fong, Galvez, Shelker, & Loo, 2018).

Ketamine is not currently considered the first option for the treatment of depression, but it is becoming more and more common for health practitioners to consider it when the most commonly prescribed pharmaceuticals do not provide adequate relief.

Ketamine works quickly, sometimes within hours of receiving treatment. When major depression is resistant to treatment, it typically means that the common drugs prescribed have not been effective. It can also take weeks to see improvements if the medicine works at all for the patient. In the meantime, many people are at risk for suicidal ideation and susceptible to the damaging effects of treatment-resistant depression.

Ketamine can improve symptoms within just a few hours of treatment, working on different receptors in the brain and possibly offering long-term relief with multiple doses over time.

Ketamine and psychotherapy

Because ketamine can allow a person to be less preoccupied with inhibitions and feel more open to a discussion, these sessions may offer a new way to approach depression therapy and more effectively address factors like previous exposure to trauma. One study about ketamine-assisted psychotherapy discusses the administration of small doses of ketamine during a talk therapy session and the benefit of that session to someone suffering from treatment-resistant depression (Dore et al., 2019). In addition, the authors document the beneficial effects of ketamine in larger doses with supportive psychotherapy for many other conditions, including PTSD, ADHD, and generalized anxiety.

Psychotherapy is a helpful treatment for depression, whether ketamine is used simultaneously to facilitate a therapy session or the treatments occur at different times. The potential benefits of ketamine can generally promote a greater sense of well-being, increasing the possibility of full participation in the therapeutic process or greater engagement with therapy on behalf of the patient.

IS KETAMINE LEGAL?

Ketamine is a legally available medicine for anesthesia and depression and is commonly used for other purposes. It is an 'essential medicine' due to its low cost and high utility, according to the World Health Organization (WHO). It is the only legal psychedelic therapy available for treating depression in the United States for most people at this time. Although legal, it remains a controlled substance and must be prescribed by a qualified clinician.

Ketamine is not legal for recreational purposes and can be dangerous if used improperly.

IS KETAMINE TREATMENT APPROVED BY THE FDA?

The FDA (U.S. Food and Drug Administration) has approved esketamine (Spravato) for the treatment of depression in conjunction with traditional antidepressants.

Use of ketamine outside the FDA-labeled indication is termed 'off-label' use. This simply means the FDA has not approved it for that purpose, although it could be quite reasonable to use it for that purpose due to supporting studies. Ketamine practitioners using higher doses or routes of administration different than those in formal clinical trials are engaging in 'off-label' use. In some cases this could be helpful and offer additional benefits, while in others it may be too experimental and carry increased risks.

IS KETAMINE FOR DEPRESSION SAFE?

It is important to know that ketamine taken in high doses is used for anesthesia purposes but does not have the same effect as subanesthetic doses used in depression.

That being said, side effects do occur with low doses administered to treat depression. Study participants have reported symptoms like feeling odd, the sensation of floating, sedation, dissociation, and impaired cognitive abilities. Physical side effects can include increased blood pressure and heart rates, dizziness, vomiting, and headaches. The long-term effects of treatment with ketamine are not currently known. Further studies are required to discover any risk of lasting impacts that could exist.

The infrequent doses are administered under the supervision of a professional in a clinical setting, followed by health monitoring and observation for a period of time after treatment. This helps ensure safety after treatment, as the common side effects can be dangerous if a person is not supervised until they subside.

Ketamine should not be taken daily and only at home under the supervision or guidance of a trained practitioner. Working with a practitioner and receiving the medicine with medical direction is the only way to be confident that treatment will be as safe as possible.

It is important to note that ketamine is commonly misused as a street drug and can have addictive properties if taken without the guidance and supervision of a practitioner. When used improperly, it has the potential to cause psychological and physical harm, such as neurocognitive problems or difficulty functioning normally and lower urinary tract symptoms, painful urination, or blood in the urine.

CAN YOU GET ADDICTED TO KETAMINE?

Ketamine is a schedule III -controlled substance in the U.S. and does carry a risk of habituation, tolerance, and addiction in recreational or unsupervised settings. However, ketamine addiction is less likely to occur when the drug is used for supervised medical treatments. This is because ketamine treatments are typically administered at lower doses and on an intermittent basis rather than continuously. Additionally, most ketamine treatments occur in a clinical setting rather than at home. As a result, patients are less likely to develop problematic patterns of use. While ketamine addiction is possible, it is less likely to occur when the drug is used for its approved medical purposes. Because of the lower dosage and intermittent use pattern of treatments, it's less likely that you'll become addicted to ketamine. Currently, most ketamine treatments occur in a clinical setting and

Always work with a practitioner who can help ensure the correct dose and frequency of ketamine and esketamine to reduce the risk of addiction or dependency. Individual use not regulated by a professional increases the likelihood of abuse, in addition to the dangers of possible side effects in a non-clinical setting.

IS KETAMINE FOR DEPRESSION COVERED BY INSURANCE?

Because ketamine is not considered the first line of defense against depression, some insurance companies will not cover it.

However, some plans will cover ketamine for depression if certain criteria are met, such as trying at least two or more medications that haven't helped at all on their own. In this case, insurance companies will likely review a case and may require the completion of prior authorization procedures.

It is always best to speak with your insurance company for information about what is covered and which steps can be taken to have treatments approved if a plan allows coverage for ketamine treatments.

WHERE CAN I FIND KETAMINE TREATMENT FOR DEPRESSION?

Ketamine has been shown to be an effective treatment for certain mental health conditions, but it is not without its risks. When misused, ketamine can lead to serious health problems, including addiction and dependence. It is not recommended that individuals acquire or use ketamine themselves, as there are serious concerns about dosage and safety that require oversight by a professional, and doing so is illegal. For this reason, it is not recommended that individuals attempt to self-medicate with ketamine. Instead, ketamine should only be used under the supervision of a trained professional. Additionally, attempts at self-medication increase the likelihood of dependency, addiction, and health risks. Ketamine, if deemed appropriate, is only one part of a treatment regimen that may require conjunctive prescription antidepressants, behavioral therapy, or other interventions and lifestyle changes for best results.

As ketamine research continues to provide a greater understanding of its effect on depression, it is becoming more widely available for therapeutic use by mental health professionals. To ensure the quality of medicine and safe use, connect with an experienced practitioner. They can provide ketamine treatment that is right for a person's individual needs.

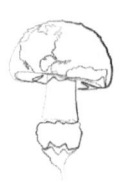

REFERENCES:

- Ansara, E. D. (2020). Management of treatment-resistant generalized anxiety disorder. *The mental health clinician, 10*(6), 326-334. doi:10.9740/mhc.2020.11.326
- Dore, J., Turnipseed, B., Dwyer, S., Turnipseed, A., Andries, J., Ascani, G., . . . Wolfson, P. (2019). Ketamine Assisted Psychotherapy (KAP): Patient Demographics, Clinical Data and Outcomes in Three Large Practices Administering Ketamine with Psychotherapy. *Journal of Psychoactive Drugs, 51*(2), 189-198. doi:10.1080/02791072.2019.1587556
- FDA. (2019). US Food and Drug Administration. FDA approves new nasal spray medication for treatment-resistant depression; available only at a certified doctor's office or clinic. *FDA Website*. Retrieved from https://www.fda.gov/news-events/press-announcements/fda-approves-new-nasal-spray-medication-

treatment-resistant-depression-available-only-certified?dom=prime&src=syn
- Serafini, G., Howland, R. H., Rovedi, F., Girardi, P., & Amore, M. (2014). The role of ketamine in treatment-resistant depression: a systematic review. *Current Neuropharmacology, 12*(5), 444-461. doi:10.2174/1570159X12666140619204251
- Short, B., Fong, J., Galvez, V., Shelker, W., & Loo, C. K. (2018). Side-effects associated with ketamine use in depression: a systematic review. *Lancet Psychiatry, 5*(1), 65-78. doi:10.1016/s2215-0366(17)30272-9
- Wilkowska, A., Szałach, Ł., & Cubała, W. J. (2020). Ketamine in Bipolar Disorder: A Review. *Neuropsychiatric disease and treatment, 16*, 2707-2717. doi:10.2147/NDT.S282208

EIGHTEEN
CAN KETAMINE THERAPY HELP WITH SUICIDAL IDEATION?
SOPHIE SAINT THOMAS

MEDICALLY REVIEWED BY DR. DAVID COX, PHD, ABPP AND DR. DAVID FLYNN, MD, MBA, CPHQ

Suicidal ideation is a troubling and painful side effect of conditions such as post-traumatic stress disorder (PTSD) or major depressive disorder. One's life becomes interrupted by violent imagery, feelings of emptiness, and in more extreme cases even detailed written plans on how they would commit suicide. However, despite this intense experience one does not necessarily want to die - instead it usually means that a person wants to live but is in need of compassionate and effective care.

Ketamine may be a promising treatment for those who suffer from suicidal ideation. It has been shown to help reduce the severity of these feelings, and because it works so quickly many people with severe depression are able to get relief within hours rather than weeks or months

WHAT IS KETAMINE?

Ketamine is currently the only legally approved psychedelic. It is FDA approved in the form of the nasal spray Spravato (esketamine), for treatment-resistant depression. While a ketamine infusion is a mixture of two mirror-image molecules, "R" and "S" ketamine, the FDA-approved nasal spray, Spravato (esketamine) only contains the "S" molecule.

Ketamine has been used as a safe and effective anesthetic for decades, dating back to the battlefields of Vietnam, but it has only recently started to gain momentum in the psychiatric community because of its therapeutic properties. Ketamine was discovered in 1956 and approved in 1970 as an anesthetic agent derived from phencyclidine. Compared to opiates, ketamine is relatively safe as both an anesthetic agent and pain-reliever in hospital patients. It maintains hemodynamic stability, or stable blood flow, which is invaluable when treating physical trauma in a battlefield or emergency room setting.

Ketamine is listed on the World Health Organization Model List of Essential Medicines, which lists drugs considered to be the most effective and safe while meeting a health system's most important needs.

Because ketamine sometimes elicits pleasurable side effects such as euphoria and relaxation, it is also a popular recreational drug. While it is regarded as a generally safe medicine when used appropriately, people seeking ketamine-assisted therapy should work closely with a qualified practitioner to avoid abuse or dependence.

SUICIDAL IDEATION EXPLAINED

Suicidal ideation is a common symptom of depression and PTSD. It doesn't have its own official diagnosis; rather, it often occurs alongside other mental health conditions such as PTSD, anxiety, or depression. Suicide is the 10th most common cause of death in the U.S. (Klonsky, May, & Saffer, 2016) and is a leading cause of death and disability worldwide (Klonsky et al., 2016). According to the CDC, even more people think about suicide than we have currently documented. While there were more than 47,500 deaths by suicide in 2019, 12 million American adults seriously thought about suicide, 3.5 million planned a suicide attempt, and 1.4 million attempted suicide.

Many of these people suffer from mental health conditions such as PTSD or depression. A 2015 study also suggests that the stigma surrounding mental illness may contribute to suicidal ideation (Oexle et al., 2017). Compassionate care focused on reducing the stigma associated with mental health could make life easier for those with mental health issues.

To make matters more complicated, the current first line of treatment for depression, such as SSRI antidepressants, doesn't work for everyone. According to a 2012 study, it is estimated that only 60-70% of people with depression experience positive results from traditional antidepressants such as SSRIs (Al-Harbi, 2012).

KETAMINE TREATMENT FOR SUICIDAL IDEATION

Intervening as soon as possible with a person who is experiencing suicidal ideation is the best course of action. While it can take up to six weeks for an SSRI drug like Prozac or Zoloft (or any other antidepressants) to start working, ketamine infusions have been shown to show significant improvement from day one. A 2017 study suggests that even a single dose of ketamine rapidly reduced suicidal thoughts within one day, and the reduction in suicidal ideation lasted for up to one week in depressed patients with suicidal ideation (Wilkinson et al., 2018). The ketamine dosage for depression is administered in subanesthetic doses, usually at 0.5

mg/kg (some patients may respond to doses as low as 0.1 mg/kg, whilst others may need up to 0.75 mg/kg).

Another 2018 study, which focused on patients with clinically significant suicidal ideation in major depressive disorder, suggests that subanesthetic intravenous ketamine significantly reduced suicidal ideation for up to six weeks (Grunebaum et al., 2018). While more research is needed to wholly grasp ketamine's mechanism of action, evidence suggests that it is multifactorial, including inhibiting the uptake of biogenic amines, inhibiting opioid receptor binding, and inhibition of N-methyl D-aspartate (NMDA) receptors (Grady, Marsh, Tenhouse, & Klein, 2018).

One effective ketamine infusion protocol is to begin an initial round of six infusions given over a two-week period. The doctor or therapist will assess the patient after three sessions to evaluate the impact. If the patient is improving, they complete the six-week course, usually feeling the benefits in hours to even days after a single infusion. Everyone is different, but after the initial six sessions, patients generally return for booster infusions as needed, perhaps once a month, or more or less frequently depending on the severity of the symptoms.

The Spravato esketamine nasal spray is the only FDA-approved ketamine treatment for mental health disorders. It has been approved as a medicine for treatment-resistant depression. However, a 2019 study suggests that ketamine infusions may reduce suicidal ideation more effectively than the nasal spray, which showed only marginal effectiveness (Witt et al., 2020). Therefore, while treatment plans should be discussed with a doctor, off-label infusions may be the most beneficial method of ketamine administration for those with suicidal thoughts.

KETAMINE MAY BE A POWERFUL TOOL IN THE MENTAL HEALTH CRISIS

Between 1999 to 2018, suicide rates in the U.S. increased by 35%. The number of deaths by suicide has climbed dramatically during the Covid-19 pandemic. It is alarmingly evident that suicide is a public health crisis, and intervention for those experiencing suicidal ideation is crucial. Traditional antidepressants such as SSRIs have a number of limitations, creating a need for new solutions. The FDA approval of the esketamine nasal spray was a landmark decision for psychedelic therapy; however, studies of off-label infusions have demonstrated even greater efficacy in the management of suicidal ideation. As a society, the U.S. needs to work to destigmatize mental health treatment, in addition to further funding the research of novel and promising treatments such as ketamine infusions.

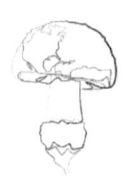

REFERENCES:

- Al-Harbi, K. S. (2012). Treatment-resistant depression: therapeutic trends, challenges, and future directions. *Patient preference and adherence, 6*, 369-388. doi:10.2147/PPA.S29716
- Grady, S. E., Marsh, T. A., Tenhouse, A., & Klein, K. (2018). Ketamine for the treatment of major depressive disorder and bipolar depression: A review of the literature. *The mental health clinician, 7*(1), 16-23. doi:10.9740/mhc.2017.01.016
- Grunebaum, M. F., Galfalvy, H. C., Choo, T. H., Keilp, J. G., Moitra, V. K., Parris, M. S., . . . Mann, J. J. (2018). Ketamine for Rapid Reduction of Suicidal Thoughts in Major

- Depression: A Midazolam-Controlled Randomized Clinical Trial. *Am J Psychiatry, 175*(4), 327-335. doi:10.1176/appi.ajp.2017.17060647
- Klonsky, E. D., May, A. M., & Saffer, B. Y. (2016). Suicide, Suicide Attempts, and Suicidal Ideation. *Annu Rev Clin Psychol, 12*, 307-330. doi:10.1146/annurev-clinpsy-021815-093204
- Oexle, N., Ajdacic-Gross, V., Kilian, R., Müller, M., Rodgers, S., Xu, Z., . . . Rüsch, N. (2017). Mental illness stigma, secrecy and suicidal ideation. *Epidemiol Psychiatr Sci, 26*(1), 53-60. doi:10.1017/s2045796015001018
- Wilkinson, S. T., Ballard, E. D., Bloch, M. H., Mathew, S. J., Murrough, J. W., Feder, A., . . . Sanacora, G. (2018). The Effect of a Single Dose of Intravenous Ketamine on Suicidal Ideation: A Systematic Review and Individual Participant Data Meta-Analysis. *Am J Psychiatry, 175*(2), 150-158. doi:10.1176/appi.ajp.2017.17040472
- Witt, K., Potts, J., Hubers, A., Grunebaum, M. F., Murrough, J. W., Loo, C., . . . Hawton, K. (2020). Ketamine for suicidal ideation in adults with psychiatric disorders: A systematic review and meta-analysis of treatment trials. *Aust N Z J Psychiatry, 54*(1), 29-45. doi:10.1177/0004867419883341

NINETEEN
KETAMINE ASSISTED PSYCHOTHERAPY
HILARY SPARROW, MA, LPC, AND MARGARET SHARPE, MSW, LCSW

MEDICALLY REVIEWED BY DR. DAVID COX, PHD, ABPP AND DR. DAVID FLYNN, MD, MBA, CPHQ

In 2019, the FDA approved ketamine for treatment-resistant depression (Swainson et al., 2019), and since then it has shown promise in combination with psychotherapy for depressive, anxious, and emotional trauma states. When used in combination with psychotherapy, ketamine can help to reduce symptoms by creating a temporary state of dissociation that allows patients to process emotions and memories without being overwhelmed by them. Since then, it has also been combined with psychotherapy to assist in symptom resolution for depressive, anxious, and emotional trauma states.

Ketamine Assisted Psychotherapy (KAP) is a technique that combines ketamine administration with a concurrent psychotherapeutic process. Ketamine dosage and method of administration vary depending on the client, psychological profile, and goals for treatment. Ketamine therapy has many treatment models and can be administered via intravenous (IV) injection, intramuscular (IM) injection, intranasal (IN) spray, sublingual, or oral administration. The amount of medicine that actually becomes available to the patient is called its bioavailability. Bioavailability varies as follows: IM/IV: ninety-three to ninety-five percent; IN and Sublingual: twenty-five to thirty percent; oral: ten percent or less (Andrade, 2017; Fanta, Kinnunen, Backman, & Kalso, 2015; Murrough et al., 2015; Rolan, Lim, Sunderland, Liu, & Molnar, 2014; Swiatek, Jordan, & Coffman, 2016). Administration can be conducted by a psychiatrist, a psychiatric nurse practitioner, or a psychotherapist working with a prescribing professional.

Research shows ketamine can enhance the process of psychotherapy (Hasler, 2020). The KAP experience provides an interruption from typical thoughts, emotions, and body sensations associated with symptoms of depression, anxiety, and other emotional distress. This is particularly useful when thoughts become rigid and ruminative to the point of dysfunction, causing distress, harm, or emotional overwhelm. Using ketamine with psychotherapy aids trauma processing by creating synaptic plasticity, facilitating fear extinction, blocking memory reconciliation, and improving the ability to process traumatic memories (Krediet et al., 2020; Myers & Davis, 2007). It provides a glimpse of what an individual may look like removed from their distressing thought narratives or behavior patterns. Ketamine treatments, combined with psychotherapy, renew possibility and hope.

Psychedelic therapies, like KAP, can increase awareness of behavioral patterns, ways of relating, and schemas that reinforce emotional distress. These therapies can augment traditional psychotherapy, allowing the client to access higher levels of fluidity, flexibility, and malleability in thought and behavioral patterns. In addition, psychedelic therapy enhances neural plasticity and can improve the therapeutic alliance by promoting feelings of openness and enhancing empathy toward self and others.

KETAMINE ASSISTED PSYCHOTHERAPY LED BY A PSYCHOTHERAPIST

Before a licensed psychotherapist can provide KAP, patients are required to have a medical evaluation with a physician, psychiatrist, or psychiatric nurse practitioner. The prescriber must establish that there is a medical need for the treatment. Then, an initial ketamine session can be conducted to ensure that the patient can tolerate the medicine safely and without any adverse reactions. There are some contraindications for KAP, such as certain medications, high blood pressure, and certain heart conditions. If there are no contraindications, the therapist will prescribe ketamine lozenges (troches) for the client to bring to the office for treatment. During the session, the client will dissolve the troche under their tongue and receive guidance and support from the therapist.

Treatments with a psychotherapist tend to involve lower doses so that the client can connect with inner experiences while also being able to maintain a dialogue with the therapist. Ketamine treatments create decreased activity within the default mode network and a reduced level of physiological activation when accessing distressing memories or emotions (Li et al., 2020). Combining psychotherapeutic techniques with ketamine accelerates the typical psychotherapy process. Interhemispheric communication often invites new insights.

KAP LOZENGE SESSION

The length of a session may vary based on the needs of the client, but most KAP sessions last up to three hours. The first thirty minutes are typically spent discussing desired outcomes and setting intentions. This is an important part of the process, as it helps to focus the session and ensure that the client's needs are met. Some clients also choose to create a ceremonial practice, such as bringing an object of personal significance to have present during the session. This can provide comfort and support during what may be a challenging experience. Next, the patient ingests the lozenge orally. Rapid-release lozenges dissolve instantly, and more traditional lozenges dissolve after about five minutes. Patients then swish the dissolved lozenge with the saliva in the mouth, allowing the medicine to be absorbed through the mucus membranes. The swishing process lasts from seven to fifteen minutes as directed by the prescriber., The longer the oral solution is in the mouth, the higher quantity of medicine is absorbed. Depending on the goals for the session, the prescriber will direct the time of the oral solution.

Patients typically swallow the medicine and lie down on a couch; adding an eye mask and noise-canceling headphones with ambient music can help direct the experience inward. This allows the patient to tend to whatever thoughts, feelings, or sensations that may show up. The client typically "peaks" at about one hour, marking the strongest point of the experience, while the second hour may include either more inward work or outward processing with the therapist, depending on the patient's needs. During the last thirty minutes, the therapist will assist the client in preparing for the conclusion of the session, offering grounding strategies like stretching, breathwork, or continued therapeutic processing.

NON-DIRECTIVE APPROACH

KAP differs from traditional clinical interventions as it uses a non-directive approach similar to the modality in MDMA protocols for treating PTSD (Michael C. Mithoefer, 2017). This modality views the client as the expert on themselves. The experience unfolds naturally as the client follows body sensations, emotions, and memories as they arise. It is a client-directed approach with the therapist following the client's lead. The client is encouraged to connect with sources of inner healing intelligence versus seeking external cues for directing their experience (for example, asking the therapist or guide). They acknowledge inward sources of validation and motivation, strengthen internal locus of control, and become the director of their healing journey. They view themselves as the authority or "expert" of themselves and their healing process versus externalizing their healing. They are encouraged to let go of the need to control and to turn off normal cognitive processes to direct awareness more into the body.

CATALYST THERAPY

KAP and other psychedelic therapies have been described as catalysts and accelerants to traditional psychotherapy processes (Vermetten et al., 2020). The psychedelic experience helps overcome barriers and resistance to typical psychotherapy limitations. Psychotherapy and the path to healing involve connecting with difficult emotions such as sadness, pain, grief, loss, devastation, and fear. Although it may be difficult, accessing, honoring, and expressing these emotions can be an antidote to suffering. Resistance to or premature discontinuation of psychotherapy often occurs as clients struggle to face difficult emotions.

KAP therapies help individuals connect with these emotions due to the pharmacological impact on the brain and memory reconsolidation. The experience facilitates processing traumatic memories with reduced physiological activation due to the reduced blood flow and connectivity in the default mode network and limbic system. Psychedelics also facilitate rapid interhemispheric communication and can aid in advanced processing, which creates an accelerant impact. This helps explain why psychedelic therapy accelerates the psychotherapeutic process.

POST-SESSION INTEGRATION

Ketamine-assisted Psychotherapy (KAP) has been shown to promote neural plasticity in order to help clients shift negative cognitive narratives, schemas, and behavior patterns. During a KAP session, clients typically experience profound insights and newfound perspectives on their lives. These insights can be extremely helpful in promoting lasting change. Following a KAP session, clients typically return for an integration session with their therapist. This provides an opportunity to process through and integrate any insights gained during the ketamine session in order to create lasting changes in alignment with healing goals. KAP, combined with integration approaches, improves emotional regulation abilities, and clients develop trust in themselves to face their world with renewed boldness, strength, and interpersonal satisfaction.

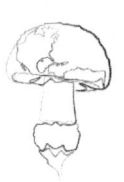

REFERENCES:

- Andrade, C. (2017). Ketamine for Depression, 4: In What Dose, at What Rate, by What Route, for How Long, and at What Frequency? *The Journal of Clinical Psychiatry, 78*(7), e852-e857. doi:10.4088/jcp.17f11738

- Fanta, S., Kinnunen, M., Backman, J. T., & Kalso, E. (2015). Population pharmacokinetics of S-ketamine and norketamine in healthy volunteers after intravenous and oral dosing. *Eur J Clin Pharmacol, 71*(4), 441-447. doi:10.1007/s00228-015-1826-y
- Hasler, G. (2020). Toward specific ways to combine ketamine and psychotherapy in treating depression. *CNS Spectr, 25*(3), 445-447. doi:10.1017/s1092852919001007
- Krediet, E., Bostoen, T., Breeksema, J., van Schagen, A., Passie, T., & Vermetten, E. (2020). Reviewing the Potential of Psychedelics for the Treatment of PTSD. *International Journal of Neuropsychopharmacology, 23*(6), 385-400. doi:10.1093/ijnp/pyaa018
- Li, M., Woelfer, M., Colic, L., Safron, A., Chang, C., Heinze, H. J., . . . Walter, M. (2020). Default mode network connectivity change corresponds to ketamine's delayed glutamatergic effects. *Eur Arch Psychiatry Clin Neurosci, 270*(2), 207-216. doi:10.1007/s00406-018-0942-y
- Michael C. Mithoefer, M. D. (2017). A Manual for MDMA-Assisted Psychotherapy in the Treatment of Posttraumatic Stress Disorder, Version 8.1: . *Multidisciplinary Association for Psychedelic Studies (MAPS)*.
- Murrough, J. W., Soleimani, L., DeWilde, K. E., Collins, K. A., Lapidus, K. A., Iacoviello, B. M., . . . Charney, D. S. (2015). Ketamine for rapid reduction of suicidal ideation: a randomized controlled trial. *Psychological medicine, 45*(16), 3571-3580. doi:10.1017/s0033291715001506
- Myers, K. M., & Davis, M. (2007). Mechanisms of fear extinction. *Molecular Psychiatry, 12*(2), 120-150. doi:10.1038/sj.mp.4001939
- Rolan, P., Lim, S., Sunderland, V., Liu, Y., & Molnar, V. (2014). The absolute bioavailability of racemic ketamine from a novel sublingual formulation. *British journal of clinical pharmacology, 77*(6), 1011-1016. doi:10.1111/bcp.12264

- Swainson, J., Thomas, R. K., Archer, S., Chrenek, C., MacKay, M. A., Baker, G., . . . Demas, M. L. (2019). Esketamine for treatment resistant depression. *Expert Rev Neurother, 19*(10), 899-911. doi:10.1080/14737175.2019.1640604
- Swiatek, K. M., Jordan, K., & Coffman, J. (2016). New use for an old drug: oral ketamine for treatment-resistant depression. *BMJ Case Rep, 2016*. doi:10.1136/bcr-2016-216088
- Vermetten, E., Krediet, E., Bostoen, T., Breeksema, J. J., Schoevers, R. A., & van den Brink, W. (2020). [Psychedelics in the treatment of PTSD]. *Tijdschr Psychiatr, 62*(8), 640-649.

PART FOUR
MAGIC MUSHROOMS (PSILOCYBIN)

"When we look within ourselves with psilocybin, we discover that we do not have to look outward toward the futile promise of life that circles distant stars in order to still our cosmic loneliness. We should look within; the paths of the heart lead to nearby universes full of life and affection for humanity."

Terence McKenna

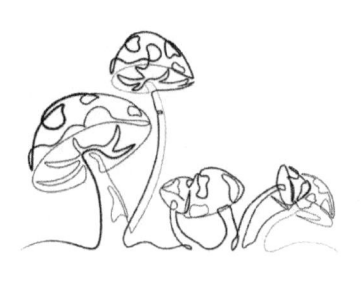

TWENTY
A BEGINNER'S GUIDE TO PSILOCYBIN
AMBER KRAUS

MEDICALLY REVIEWED BY DR. DAVID COX, PHD, ABPP

Psilocybin is a naturally occurring psychoactive compound that can be found in over 200 species of mushrooms. While its chemical structure closely resembles serotonin, the effects of psilocybin are dramatically different. Ingesting "magic mushrooms" derived from this species of fungi can provide intense spiritual and mystical experiences. These profound effects have led to increased popularity of psilocybin in recent years. Despite its potential medicinal and therapeutic benefits, psilocybin is currently classified as a Schedule I drug and is illegal in the United States and most other countries. However, continued scientific research on the effects of psilocybin may eventually change its legal status.

WHAT ARE MAGIC MUSHROOMS?

"Magic mushrooms" are a type of mushroom that contains psilocybin, and this psychedelic substance gives magic mushrooms their hallucinogenic effects. Magic mushrooms can be found in different parts of the world, including Mexico, Asia, and Australia.

They typically grow out of decomposing matter, such as dung or wood chips.

Psilocybin has a long history of therapeutic use and has been used by indigenous cultures for thousands of years. This psychedelic drug was used for healing, spiritual and religious ceremonies, and other purposes by many ancient cultures in Central and South America. It wasn't until the 1950s that psilocybin gained notoriety in modern Western medicine when the businessman and scientist R. Gordon Wasson brought psilocybin mushrooms back from a trip to Mexico. He shared a sample with scientist Albert Hofmann—also known for discovering the psychedelic properties of LSD—who was able to isolate the psychedelic compound in the mushrooms. Since then, numerous studies have been done on the effects of psilocybin and its potential medicinal and therapeutic benefits.

The term "magic mushroom" gained mainstream popularity after the 1957 release of a *Life* Magazine article entitled "Seeking the Magic Mushroom," in which Wasson recounted his experiences with the substance.

PSILOCYBIN'S INTERACTION WITH THE BODY AND BRAIN

The compound works by stimulating serotonin levels in the brain. Serotonin is a hormone that is responsible for regulating mood, feelings of well-being, and happiness. Psilocybin has been studied as a treatment for anxiety and depression because serotonin levels play a key role in mood disorders (Johnson & Griffiths, 2017). The results of studies on the efficacy of psilocybin as a treatment for anxiety and depression have been mixed. Some studies have found that psilocybin can reduce symptoms of anxiety and depression, while other studies have found no significant effects. Despite the mixed results, psilocybin research is ongoing, and the compound holds promise as a treatment for mood disorders.

So, what does a magic mushroom trip feel like? Psilocybin mushrooms are hallucinogenic that affect the brain's prefrontal cortex. The prefrontal cortex is responsible for abstract thinking, thought analysis, mood, and perception, among other things. And while outcomes will be different for each user based on their body chemistry as well as mindset and the setting in which the drugs are taken, studies, as well as anecdotal data, suggests that many users report feelings of euphoria and even transcendence or mystical experiences. Colors and sounds may appear sharpened or heightened as one begins to notice changes in perception of their surroundings. Users may begin to feel a sense of openness and connection to the world, as well as a strong connection to their thoughts and feelings.

It is possible, though unlikely in most cases, to have a "bad trip" while under the influence of psilocybin mushrooms. While the idea of openness and feelings of connection to one's thoughts and feelings may seem like a good thing, it can also lead to increased feelings of anxiety or intense reactions to one's thoughts.

The long-term effects of psilocybin use are still being studied and require more research. A 2020 study published in *Scientific Reports* indicated that the positive effects of psilocybin lasted for up to one month after users were given a single dose of psilocybin (Barrett, Doss, Sepeda, Pekar, & Griffiths, 2020). The study indicated that emotions and brain function as a response to both positive and negative stimuli were altered long after the psilocybin had left the user's body. Elsewhere, even longer post-treatment improvement has been reported (Johnson, Garcia-Romeu, Cosimano, & Griffiths, 2014). This is an indicator that psilocybin mushrooms could have long-term benefits for those interested in treating mood disorders.

BENEFITS OF PSILOCYBIN

Studies by Johns Hopkins Medicine show that ingesting psilocybin alongside psychotherapy significantly reduced symptoms in people with major depressive disorder and relieved anxiety and depression in those with end-of-life cancer diagnoses (Davis et al., 2021). Moreover, these studies showed that depression symptoms were relieved more quickly than by other treatments for depression. One study showed that 67% of participants showed more than a 50% reduction in symptoms after just one week. This number increased to 71% of participants after four weeks.

There is limited research on the effects of psilocybin as a treatment for alcohol misuse, although some studies have shown promising results and justify the need for funding to conduct larger clinical trials (Johnson & Griffiths, 2017). Similarly, limited studies have been done on the use of psilocybin for treatment-resistant tobacco and nicotine dependence (Johnson et al., 2014). The results were similar to those of the alcohol-dependence studies and indicated promising results that warrant additional research (Bogenschutz et al., 2015).

HOW TO TAKE PSILOCYBIN

There are several different ways to ingest mushrooms. Some people choose to eat them whole, although the general opinion is that they don't taste great. To mask the taste, other options are to grind the dried mushrooms and blend them into smoothies or juices, or even place the ground mushrooms into capsules. Another option is to brew the mushrooms into tea and drink it. Drinking a mushroom tea will bring on the effects the quickest and ingesting a capsule will take the longest for effects to show up.

Before taking magic mushrooms, a user should make sure to have plenty of time set aside. The effects of psilocybin can usually be felt for up to six hours, with the peak happening around 2-3 hours after ingestion. If a user has never taken mushrooms before, they should leave the whole day free of responsibilities to ensure ample time for recovery.

It is also important to take the proper dose. A first-time user should start with a small dose. In clinical settings, a common dose ranges from 15-30 mg. More experienced users may choose to increase the dosage but starting with a low dose is a safer decision.

WHAT TO EXPECT ON A MAGIC MUSHROOM TRIP

When psilocybin is ingested, it causes a range of perceptual changes, including visual halos around lights and objects, vivid colors, distorted vision, emotional shifts, and a distorted sense of time (Passie, Seifert, Schneider, & Emrich, 2002). Users may also experience heightened thoughts and emotions. One may feel more connected to nature or the universe, their loved ones, and oneself. Many users report feeling a sense of peace and openness.

Physical side effects can vary from person to person. Some users report feeling nauseous in the first 60-90 minutes after ingestion, although ingesting the mushrooms in tea form may reduce nausea. Additional physical symptoms may include changes in heart rate or blood pressure, restlessness or arousal, or trouble with coordination (Hasler, Grimberg, Benz, Huber, & Vollenweider, 2004).

HOW LONG WILL A TRIP LAST?

A magic mushroom trip typically lasts somewhere between 4-6 hours, with the peak of the trip occurring 2-3 hours after ingestion. In the first hour or so of the trip, some users may have mild feelings of anxiety and may wonder if the mushrooms are providing the intended effects. It is important not to take an additional dose, as this may lead to unintended results. During the peak of the trip is when a user will feel the most intense sensory and psychological alterations. This is a good time to relax and lean into whatever feelings or perceptions may arise. As users begin to come down from the trip, they are likely to experience a gradual decrease in effects.

The day after a trip may leave users feeling tired. In the days and even weeks after a trip, one may still feel some lasting effects, including improved mood and openness to others. The effects of a magic mushroom trip may even last for years. In a study at Johns Hopkins Medical Center, 94% of patients who took psilocybin reported the experience to be "one of the top five most meaningful experiences of their lives." Furthermore, the friends, family members, and colleagues of the patients also reported noticing that the patients were happier, calmer, and kinder—even after 14 months (Griffiths, Richards, Johnson, McCann, & Jesse, 2008).

RISKS AND POSSIBLE SIDE EFFECTS

Research continues on the benefits, risks, and possible side effects of psilocybin use. A 2010 study analyzed data gathered from eight double-blind placebo-controlled studies conducted between 1999 and 2008 that included 110 healthy subjects who received oral doses of psilocybin (Studerus, Kometer, Hasler, & Vollenweider, 2010). The analysis found that dysphoria, anxiety, and panic occurred only in the two highest dose conditions, and even then, only in a small number of subjects. Most patients in the studies reported pleasant experiences. The analysis found that "the administration of moderate doses of psilocybin to healthy, high-functioning, and well-prepared subjects in the context of a carefully monitored research environment is associated with an acceptable level of risk."

Even in uncontrolled, recreational settings, anecdotal data suggests that most experiences with psilocybin are positive and produce little to no long-term negative effects. When taking psilocybin recreationally and in a non-clinical setting, finding a safe and comfortable setting reduces the risk of experiencing a bad trip.

CAN YOU OVERDOSE ON MAGIC MUSHROOMS?

More research needs to be done before a definitive answer can be concluded, but according to the Drug Policy Alliance, the "risk of fatal overdose is virtually non-existent." Another study indicates that there are very low rates of abuse and no potential for physical dependence.

PSILOCYBIN: A JOURNEY WITH MAGIC MUSHROOMS

Among all the psychedelics, mushrooms are perhaps the safest and most well-tolerated. Nevertheless, it is always important to take the time to prepare oneself for a psychedelic experience and respect the process. This means setting aside some time in a comfortable environment where you feel safe and relaxed. It is also advisable to have a trusted friend or therapist present to provide support if needed. When using psilocybin for medicinal purposes, it is worthwhile to have access to a trained psychotherapist who can provide guidance and support. With proper preparation and support, mushrooms can be a powerful tool for healing and self-discovery.

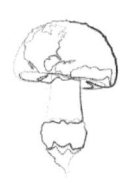

REFERENCES:

- Barrett, F. S., Doss, M. K., Sepeda, N. D., Pekar, J. J., & Griffiths, R. R. (2020). Emotions and brain function are altered up to one month after a single high dose of psilocybin. *Scientific Reports, 10*(1), 2214. doi:10.1038/s41598-020-59282-y
- Bogenschutz, M. P., Forcehimes, A. A., Pommy, J. A., Wilcox, C. E., Barbosa, P. C., & Strassman, R. J. (2015). Psilocybin-assisted treatment for alcohol dependence: a proof-of-concept study. *Journal of psychopharmacology (Oxford, England), 29*(3), 289-299. doi:10.1177/0269881114565144
- Davis, A. K., Barrett, F. S., May, D. G., Cosimano, M. P., Sepeda, N. D., Johnson, M. W., . . . Griffiths, R. R. (2021). Effects of Psilocybin-Assisted Therapy on Major Depressive Disorder: A Randomized Clinical Trial. *JAMA Psychiatry, 78*(5), 481-489. doi:10.1001/jamapsychiatry.2020.3285
- Griffiths, R., Richards, W., Johnson, M., McCann, U., & Jesse, R. (2008). Mystical-type experiences occasioned by psilocybin mediate the attribution of personal meaning and spiritual significance 14 months later. *Journal of psychopharmacology (Oxford, England), 22*(6), 621-632. doi:10.1177/0269881108094300
- Hasler, F., Grimberg, U., Benz, M. A., Huber, T., & Vollenweider, F. X. (2004). Acute psychological and physiological effects of psilocybin in healthy humans: a

double-blind, placebo-controlled dose-effect study. *Psychopharmacology (Berl), 172*(2), 145-156. doi:10.1007/s00213-003-1640-6
- Johnson, M. W., Garcia-Romeu, A., Cosimano, M. P., & Griffiths, R. R. (2014). Pilot study of the 5-HT2AR agonist psilocybin in the treatment of tobacco addiction. *Journal of psychopharmacology (Oxford, England), 28*(11), 983-992. doi:10.1177/0269881114548296
- Johnson, M. W., & Griffiths, R. R. (2017). Potential Therapeutic Effects of Psilocybin. *Neurotherapeutics : the journal of the American Society for Experimental NeuroTherapeutics, 14*(3), 734-740. doi:10.1007/s13311-017-0542-y
- Studerus, E., Kometer, M., Hasler, F., & Vollenweider, F. X. (2010). Acute, subacute and long-term subjective effects of psilocybin in healthy humans: a pooled analysis of experimental studies. *Journal of Psychopharmacology, 25*(11), 1434-1452. doi:10.1177/0269881110382466

TWENTY-ONE
HOW TO MICRODOSE WITH PSILOCYBIN MUSHROOMS
LEIA FRIEDWOMAN, MS

MEDICALLY REVIEWED BY DR. BENJAMIN MALCOLM, PHARMD, MPH, BCPP

Microdosing is a rising trend in the world of psychedelic drugs. A microdose is a sub-perceptual amount of a psychedelic drug, which means that it is an amount that does not produce any hallucinations or other perceptual changes. Initially popularized by James Fadiman in The Psychedelic Explorer's Guide, microdosing is a rising trend both in persons that want to boost productivity and creativity as well as those attempting to heal mental illness.

Microdosing has become increasingly popular in recent years as people look for ways to enhance their cognitive performance without interrupting their daily lives. Unlike larger doses of psychedelics, which can produce profound changes in consciousness, microdoses are designed to be taken without producing any acute effects. However, while a person on a microdose may not feel any immediate changes, there is some evidence that they can experience subtle changes in perception and thinking. In addition, taking even a small amount too much may result in uncomfortable emotional effects. As a result, it is important to be careful when experimenting with microdoses of psychedelics.

IS THERE RESEARCH TO SUPPORT THE EFFICACY OF MICRODOSING?

While there is still much unknown about **microdosing**, the evidence that does exist suggests that it may be a promising method for treating a variety of conditions. Currently, most research on microdosing is based on surveys and anecdotal reports, which can be subject to the placebo effect or expectation bias. Indeed, a couple of studies of microdosing have made the argument that microdosing leverages the placebo effect (Polito & Stevenson, 2019; Szigeti et al., 2021). More research is needed to determine the long-term effects of microdosing.

The Journal of Psychopharmacology published a survey study that found that out of over 1,102 people surveyed, more than half felt that microdosing helped with their mental health (Lea et al., 2020). Another survey study found that current and former microdosers scored lower on measures of dysfunctional attitudes and negative emotionality and scored higher on wisdom, open-mindedness, and creativity when compared to non-microdosing controls. Yet another study found that microdosers reported increased focus and energy (Anderson et al., 2019). These results suggest that microdosing mushrooms merits further study and may offer some people the potential to improve their mental health.

While many report reductions of anxiety or depression with microdosing, almost as many others have reported worsening of these problems or other effects such as physiological discomfort, impaired focus or energy, or difficulty thinking (Anderson et al., 2019). Some have also reported 'psychedelic' type effects such as distortions to thoughts or perceptions and more adverse types of outcomes such as panic attacks. Interestingly, one study found that despite short-term decreases in depression or anxiety, participants displayed increased neuroticism or sensitivity to negative feelings (Polito & Stevenson, 2019).

IS THERE ANYONE WHO SHOULDN'T TRY MICRODOSING?

While there is some evidence that microdosing may be helpful for people with anxiety or depression, there is very little research on the safety and efficacy of this practice in people with bipolar disorder or psychotic illness. Given the lack of data, it is not known whether microdosing is compatible with traditional treatments for these conditions. However, given the relative safety of psilocybin, it is unlikely that physical harms such as serotonin syndrome are a concern. Nonetheless, more research is needed to determine the potential risks and benefits of microdosing for people with mental illness, and it is generally advised that those with bipolar disorder or psychotic illness should avoid the use of psychedelics altogether.

IS IT LEGAL TO BUY PSILOCYBIN MUSHROOMS FOR MICRODOSING?

The illegality of psilocybin mushrooms can make it hard to access a quality product. Some people take the risk and grow their own at home, as psilocybin spores can be legally purchased online in most states, and the rest of the necessary ingredients are relatively easy to acquire. Instructions for growing psychedelic mushrooms can be found on the internet. Keep in mind that although the spores are legally available for microscopy purposes, it is illegal to use them with the intention of growing the mushrooms.

Although possession of psilocybin-containing mushrooms is illegal at the federal level, several municipalities have decriminalized psilocybin mushrooms and other naturally occurring psychedelics. Decriminalization can be a confusing term; in short, police are instructed to make enforcement a low-level priority. In some cities and states, possessing and using small amounts of psilocybin mushrooms will not result in a felony charge or potential jail time but rather a citation, similar to a parking ticket. Check the laws of your location to find out more. Even in cities and states with decriminalization of magic mushrooms, it is illegal to sell them, and federal officers can still prosecute cases.

STRATEGIES FOR MICRODOSING

There are two main ways to microdose: on an as-needed basis or on a set schedule. People who microdose "as-needed" have a sense of how a microdose affects their system, and so they use it in specific situations to accentuate the desired effects.

Two common set schedule approaches are the Fadiman Protocol and the Stamets Stack. Consumers should take note that no formal scientific research exists to validate either of these protocols, and both Fadiman and Stamets have 'skin in the game' via book sales and supplement sales, respectively.

> **The Fadiman Protocol:** Originated by Jim Fadiman, this protocol involves a three-day cycle (Fadiman, 2011). Many microdosers keep a journal to track their progress and record daily variables such as anxiety level, appetite, mood, quality of sleep, etc. Taking note of these variables could help determine whether microdosing is appropriate for you.
> The first day is the microdose day, on which you ingest your microdose and observe what happens. Look out for changes in attitude, energy, creativity, mood, and anything else that arises. The second day is a transition day where some people report an afterglow effect from the day before. Take time to notice any subtle shifts. Journaling, making art, meditating, engaging in physical activity, and talking to a friend or therapist are all ways to process and integrate the day before. Day three is an ordinary day; step back and notice

the differences between days. Day four is the next dose day. Many people continue the cycle for one to two months and then take a break for two to four weeks between cycles. Taking breaks is important due to the lack of long-term research into the effects of psychedelics and some concern for the development of cardiac valve toxicity with consistent or long-term use.

The Stamets' Stack: This protocol involves supplementing your microdose with lion's mane mushroom (50-200 mg) and niacin (100-200 mg) (Rootman et al., 2021). Mycologist Paul Stamets believes that this combination synergizes to promote neurogenesis, the formation of new neurons in the brain.

Lion's mane (*hericium erinaceus*) is an edible and medicinal mushroom that may improve mood, enhance focus, and support brain health. Stamets says that the addition of niacin assists in deliverability throughout the body. Some people experience uncomfortable warming and reddening of the skin, a side effect of niacin caused by the widening of blood vessels.

With this protocol, you microdose for four consecutive days, followed by a three-day break. Continue the four-day-on/three-day-off cycle for one month, then stop your microdosing routine for 2-4 weeks to notice any changes and allow your body to reset.

HOW TO MICRODOSE WITH PSILOCYBIN MUSHROOMS

The first step is to establish an intention. Why are you microdosing psilocybin? Remember, intentions should be flexible enough to allow for the results to emerge in their own way. Sometimes, especially after reading anecdotal reports online, people have expectations about how it should work for them. This can lead to disappointment and can take attention away from what is actually coming up in the microdosing experience. Consider finding a peer group, coach, or therapist who is experienced with microdosing phenomena and can help you on your journey. While microdoses may not produce 'full-blown' psychedelic effects, they may subtly sensitize a person to their environmental surroundings or internal emotional content. Therefore, treating microdosing with similar intentionality, support, and complementary modalities to psychedelic-assisted therapy is likely to produce the best results. In other words, the set and setting still matter even though the doses are small.

Once you have decided on a protocol to use, it's time to prepare your doses. A great way to have consistent microdoses is to use a coffee grinder to powder the dried mushrooms. While many users online purport that caps contain more psilocybin than stems, there is no research to substantiate this claim. It is true that some mushrooms may simply be more potent than others; therefore, creating a more homogenous mixture is the best way to minimize variability between doses.

How much is a microdose of psilocybin mushrooms? For most people, a microdose is about 50-250mg (0.05-0.25g) of dried mushrooms. To measure out a microdose, you'll need a jewelry scale that can measure in milligrams. If you are new to microdosing, try starting at the lower end of this range. Over time, you can experiment with what works best for your intentions. Taking note of your experience while microdosing could help determine the appropriate dose for you.

The microdose can be ingested in a gelatin capsule or mixed with food or drink like a smoothie. Some people experience nausea if they take the microdose on an empty stomach, while others find that an empty stomach works better for them since food can slow absorption. Many people find that the microdose increases their energy levels, so it's recommended to take it in the morning or at least 6-8 hours before you would want to fall asleep.

MICRODOSING PSILOCYBIN: IS IT FOR YOU?

Microdosing of psychedelics is a growing trend, but there is little clinical research to support its efficacy or safety. Some psychedelic researchers have expressed concern about the lack of data and made valid critiques of the microdosing trend. Without much clinical evidence to guide them, people who are considering microdosing are taking a risk. It may be safer to attempt microdosing under the supervision and guidance of an experienced professional who can help assess the potential benefits and risks. Tracking your experience and working with a skilled professional can help reduce risk and ensure the best results.

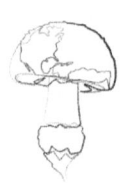

REFERENCES:

- Anderson, T., Petranker, R., Christopher, A., Rosenbaum, D., Weissman, C., Dinh-Williams, L. A., . . . Hapke, E. (2019). Psychedelic microdosing benefits and challenges: an empirical codebook. *Harm Reduct J, 16*(1), 43. doi:10.1186/s12954-019-0308-4
- Fadiman, J. (2011). *The psychedelic explorer's guide: Safe, therapeutic, and sacred journeys*: Simon and Schuster.
- Lea, T., Amada, N., Jungaberle, H., Schecke, H., Scherbaum, N., & Klein, M. (2020). Perceived outcomes of psychedelic microdosing as self-managed therapies for

mental and substance use disorders. *Psychopharmacology, 237*(5), 1521-1532. doi:10.1007/s00213-020-05477-0
- Polito, V., & Stevenson, R. J. (2019). A systematic study of microdosing psychedelics. *PloS one, 14*(2), e0211023-e0211023. doi:10.1371/journal.pone.0211023
- Rootman, J. M., Kryskow, P., Harvey, K., Stamets, P., Santos-Brault, E., Kuypers, K. P. C., . . . Walsh, Z. (2021). Adults who microdose psychedelics report health-related motivations and lower levels of anxiety and depression compared to non-microdosers. *Sci Rep, 11*(1), 22479. doi:10.1038/s41598-021-01811-4
- Szigeti, B., Kartner, L., Blemings, A., Rosas, F., Feilding, A., Nutt, D. J., . . . Erritzoe, D. (2021). Self-blinding citizen science to explore psychedelic microdosing. *Elife, 10*. doi:10.7554/eLife.62878

PART FIVE
AYAHUASCA

"Ayahuasca is a symbiotic ally of the human species."

Dennis McKenna

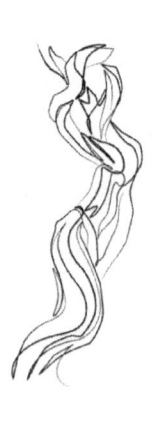

TWENTY-TWO
A BEGINNER'S GUIDE TO AYAHUASCA
LEIA FRIEDWOMAN, MS AND MAGS TANEV, MA

MEDICALLY REVIEWED BY DR. DAVID COX, PHD, ABPP

Ayahuasca is a plant-based psychedelic brew or tea with a long history of traditional use in some parts of the Amazon basin and Central America. The name ayahuasca comes from the Quechua language of the central Andes mountains, where it means "vine of the soul" or "vine of the dead." Today, ayahuasca is used by more than 75 indigenous tribes in the Amazon region for medicinal, social, religious, and spiritual purposes. Some of these communities have been engaging in the ritual use of ayahuasca for thousands of years.

When consumed, ayahuasca produces powerful psychedelic effects, including visual and auditory hallucinations, altered states of consciousness, and feelings of euphoria. For many people who drink ayahuasca, the experience is deeply meaningful and transformative.

In recent years, ayahuasca has become increasingly popular outside of its traditional cultural context, with people from all over the world traveling to participate in ceremonial sessions led by indigenous shamans or western facilitators.

Researchers have found that a single ayahuasca ceremony can have a rapid antidepressant effect (Palhano-Fontes et al., 2019) and a literature review found that ayahuasca use is safe and can be beneficial under certain conditions (Barbosa, Mizumoto, Bogenschutz, & Strassman, 2012). More research is needed in this area, especially experimental research that would control for bias, placebo, and other possible variables.

This ancient tradition is now undergoing a surge in popularity as increasing numbers of westerners seek out ayahuasca ceremonies in hopes of improved mental and/or physical health.

HOW DOES AYAHUASCA WORK?

The ayahuasca tea is brewed from two or more plants, typically the ayahuasca vine (*banisteriopsis caapi*) and chacruna leaf (*psychotria viridis*). The banisteriopsis caapi vine and the chacruna leaf do not necessarily produce a strong hallucinogenic effect on their own. When combined, these two plants result in what can be a powerful physical, emotional, and spiritual experience.

The vine contains harmala alkaloids which act as a monoamine oxidase inhibitor (MAOI), allowing for the oral absorption of dimethyltryptamine (DMT) contained in the leaves of the chacruna plant. Without the MAOI, an enzyme in the gut known as monoamine oxidase would metabolize the DMT before absorption could occur.

What happens during a ceremony can vary greatly, depending on the facilitation by the curandero or healer, the setting, the ingredients in the brew, the person's unique physiology, and more. An ayahuasca ceremony can last from 6 to 10 hours. The short-term physiological effects of ayahuasca may include nausea, vomiting, diarrhea, sweating, increased blood pressure, shaking, chills, and other physical sensations.

The psychological effects of ayahuasca can be profound and may include mystical experiences, visions, and intense emotions. Some of the more difficult psychological effects of ayahuasca, such as feeling anxiety and fear, may seem more like a nightmare than a dream. However, these challenging experiences can also provide valuable insights into one's personal psyche.

Anecdotal reports describe encounters with animals, plants, spirits, aliens, demons, and entities, as well as visiting other realms, recalling experiences from one's life in a new light, and a vast range of emotions. Ultimately, the psychological effects of ayahuasca are highly individual and dependent on factors such as set and setting, intention, and previous experience.

Ayahuasca is typically consumed in a ceremonial setting, at night, with the journeyers in the care of a trained healer (in the Shipibo lineage, curanderos go through ten years or more of rigorous training and experience). After drinking the tea, participants may experience physical, mental, emotional, and visual changes, which can induce feelings ranging from euphoria and gratitude to terror and fear.

Purging is a common aspect of the ayahuasca experience. A purge could mean vomiting, diarrhea, gas, sweating, crying, burping, yawning, shaking, laughing, and/or other vocalizing. While some sources regard these as side effects, traditional cultures believe purging is a healing component of the ayahuasca experience, as it is seen as negative energies exiting the body.

GETTING READY FOR AYAHUASCA

Proper preparation for an ayahuasca journey will ensure the best results. While specific diets vary from culture to culture, there are some commonalities. Essentially, the recommendation is to stick to clean, nutrient-dense, non-processed food and drinks. It is common practice for people to abstain from pork, cannabis, recreational drugs, and sexual activity for two weeks before and after ayahuasca. Consider avoiding caffeine, alcohol, cacao, spicy foods, dairy products, red meat, and refined sugar for at least a week leading up to the ceremony. Ripened fruit and vegetables, aged cheese, yogurt, fermented foods, yeast, and some legumes contain tyramine which can lead to medical complications when combined with ayahuasca, so these should not be eaten for at least two days before and after the ceremony. While you may not want to go into the ceremony with a completely empty stomach (you may need that energy later in the night), eat lightly. Fruits, vegetables, and some easily digestible carbohydrates are good choices. Your last meal before the ceremony should be at least four hours before.

Some medications should be discontinued for two weeks or more before an ayahuasca experience. This table, adapted from chapter 22 of the Handbook of Medical Hallucinogens and written by Kelan Thomas and Benjamin Malcolm, details a number of possible drug contraindications (Grob & Grigsby, 2021).

Potential Adverse-Drug Interactions Between Monoamine Oxidase Inhibitors (MAOIs) and Ayahuasca

Antidepressants

Selective Serotonin Reuptake Inhibitors (SSRIs)

- Celexa (Citralopram)
- Lexapro (Escitalopram)
- Paxil (Paroxetine)
- Prozac (Fluoxetine)
- Vilazodone (Vibryyd)
- Vortioxetine (Trintelix)
- Zoloft (Sertraline)

Selective Norepinephrine Reuptake Inhibitors (SNRIs)

- Cymbalta (Duloxetine)
- Effexor (Venlafaxine)
- Fetzima (Levomilnacipran)
- Pristiq (Desvenlafaxine)

Tricyclic Antidepressants

- Anadranil (Clomipramine)
- Tofranil (Imipramine)

Allergy, cough, and cold

- Chlorpheniramine
- Robitussin (Dexteromethorphan)
- Sudafed (Pseudoephedrine)

Appetite suppressants

- Adipex (Phentermine)
- Caffeine (high doses)
- Coca of cocaine
- Ephedra (*Ma Huang*)

Stimulants

- ADHD/hyperactivity stimulants
- Caffeine (high doses)
- Cocaine
- Methamphetamine
- Tobacco (oral or rectal routes)

Opioid Analgesics

- Meperidine
- Methadone
- Propoxyphene
- Tapentadol
- Tramadol

Phenethylamines

- Cathinones (mephedrone, methylenedioxypyrovalerone, and methylone)
- 2Cx, Dox, and NBOMe analogues
- MDMA
- Mescaline
- MPDV

Antipsychotics

- Ziprasidone

Mood stabalizer

- Lithium

Migraine

- Ergotamine
- Triptans

Other

- 5-HTP
- *Kambo*
- L-tryptophan
- St. John's Wort
- Trazodone

*This list is not be all-inclusive. Before consuming any medication or psychedelic, please consult with a medical professional. Most drugs listed are contraindicated due to the risk of severe serotonin toxicity while some may cause a hypertensive crisis or extreme vasoconstriction.

For those taking selective serotonin reuptake inhibitors (SSRIs), most retreat centers advise that you discontinue taking them at least six weeks before the experience (Callaway & Grob, 1998). Combining SSRIs with ayahuasca can induce serotonin syndrome, with potentially fatal effects (Domínguez-Clavé et al., 2016; Hamill, Hallak, Dursun, & Baker, 2019). Other MAO inhibiting medications should also be discontinued for at least six weeks. Please do not attempt to taper off a psychiatric medication without consulting a medical professional for safety and support.

Herbal supplements, including St. Johns Wort, Kava, or Kratom, are also something to be careful with. It is recommended that you disclose all supplements to your retreat center so that they can advise about if and how long they need to be discontinued before the ceremony.

A LOOK INSIDE AN AYAHUASCA CEREMONY

Ayahuasca ceremonies can vary wildly across different indigenous cultures, retreat centers, and facilitators. As ayahuasca has become increasingly well-known and sought after in western society, there has been a surge of neo-shamanic practitioners and other new-age healers. These practitioners may serve the medicine and conduct ceremonies with their own rituals, which often vary greatly from traditional ceremonies held by indigenous shamanic healers.

The ceremony typically takes place at night. In the traditional setting, participants gather in a maloca, an indigenous hut that's unique to tribes of the Amazon region. Participants gather at some point after nightfall and find their place in the room. Each person should have their own space, commonly a mattress on the floor where they can sit or lie down for the experience and be accompanied by their own bucket in case they need to vomit.

The person(s) serving the ayahuasca may do some sort of preparatory ritual in the space. When it is time for participants to drink the brew, they will be called up to the healer one at a time. The healer will pour the ayahuasca, possibly blessing the cup, and hand it to the person. After drinking, each participant returns to their place and gets settled in for the journey.

In some traditions, the healer will sing icaros during the ceremony. These are traditional Amazonian songs that call upon the spirit of other plants to aid in the healing of ayahuasca. In the Santo Daime tradition, the participants sing and sometimes even dance together. Some modern ceremonies include the use of live music or prerecorded instrumental music, even electronic music or some combination.

The short-term physiological effects of ayahuasca typically begin 30-60 minutes after consuming the brew. Nausea, vomiting, diarrhea, sweating, increased blood pressure, shaking, chills, crying, and emotional and perceptual changes are all commonly reported effects of the tea (Guimarães dos Santos, 2013).

The purge, described earlier, is a common occurrence in ayahuasca ceremonies. Although many westerners may have negative associations with vomiting, diarrhea, and even crying, the purge is regarded as a cleansing and healing aspect of the ayahuasca experience.

The healer/ceremony facilitator should be attentive to the physical, spiritual, energetic, and emotional state of each person in the ceremony. They may come around the room or have people come up to them to offer individual healing. Many settings also include helpers who are experienced with ayahuasca to help guide people to the bathroom, keep watch for anyone who might need attention and ensure the physical safety of everyone in the space.

After several hours, the ceremony will draw to a close. The healer may offer a closing prayer or ritual or may simply complete what they are doing and quietly leave.

IS AYAHUASCA SAFE FOR EVERYONE?

While ayahuasca has been shown to offer deep and profound healing for many people, it is not necessarily safe for everyone.

People who are affected by or have family histories of psychotic or bipolar illnesses should generally avoid the use of psychedelics.

Many facilitators and retreat centers advise that ayahuasca is contraindicated with borderline personality disorder, bipolar disorder, or schizophrenia.

For those who do choose to try ayahuasca, it is important to work with a reputable shaman or facilitator who can create a safe and supportive space. It is also important to be honest about your mental health history and any medications you are taking.

Some therapists and medical professionals advise that a person with post-traumatic stress disorder (PTSD) should proceed carefully with ayahuasca and other psychedelics, as the experience could be re-traumatizing. That being said, many people with PTSD have reported profound changes in their life, which they attribute to ayahuasca healing. Taking proper precautions, spending time to prepare, working with a skilled and experienced facilitator, keeping your expectations in check, and integrating the experience afterward can reduce the risk of adverse experiences.

Ayahuasca may not be safe for people with heart or liver problems, kidney disorders, high blood pressure, and diabetes. Someone with a serious cardiovascular disorder may be harmed by the increase in blood pressure that ayahuasca can cause.

As described earlier, certain medications, such as SSRIs, are unsafe to combine with ayahuasca.

In the Colombian yagé tradition, women on their period are not allowed under any circumstances to partake in the ceremony. The rules around this are looser in other countries.

IS AYAHUASCA LEGAL?

The answer is complicated. Ayahuasca is illegal in most countries because it contains the psychedelic dimethyltryptamine (DMT).

In the United States, ayahuasca is federally illegal as a Schedule 1 controlled substance. The Religious Freedom and Restoration Act in 1993 set a precedent that religious organizations and churches for whom ayahuasca is a sacrament *may be exempt* from legal recourse for serving the brew at their ceremonies. These exemptions are handled on a case-by-case basis; therefore, institutions that drink ayahuasca as a religious practice and/or belong to a church are not automatically exempt from the laws prohibiting ayahuasca in the U.S. The only ayahuasca churches in the U.S. with federal exemption are The União do Vegetal (UDV) and the Santo Daime church.

Ayahuasca is legal under cultural patrimony in Peru and is served in many countries in South and Central America that have a legal gray area. Some cities and states in the U.S. and countries such as Portugal have decriminalized either all drugs or at least plant-based psychedelics. However, decriminalization is not the same as legalization, and local law does not supersede federal law.

Since no jurisdiction can make a law that contradicts federal law, using the term "decriminalization" is inaccurate. A more appropriate term would be deprioritization, meaning that the local government has agreed that ayahuasca and other plant-based psychedelics should be the lowest priority of law enforcement to the police. The transport and sale of ayahuasca is seen as drug trafficking and can result in serious repercussions.

CAN YOU DIE FROM TAKING AYAHUASCA?

A number of people have died while taking ayahuasca. However, it is suspected that in the vast majority of these cases, the user died because of co-ingestion of contraindicated drugs or medications or because the ceremony environment was not safe. The estimated lethal dose of ayahuasca is approximately 20x the usual dose, which is almost impossible to ingest because vomiting would limit how much a person could consume.

Some people encounter death-like experiences while in a ceremony with ayahuasca. Understandably, this can be very frightening. Journeyers can also experience ego death or a dissolution of the sense of self.

If you find yourself in such a circumstance where you seem to no longer know who you are, try to remember that you have taken a substance, trust that you are in a process and the experience is likely to pass in a few hours. Although ego death and other transcendental experiences can be frightening and confusing at the time, it may make sense when the journey is over. If symptoms such as derealization, extreme confusion, mania, psychosis, or other concerning phenomena persist for several hours after the ceremony has drawn to a close, seek out a helper or facilitator to determine if you may need medical attention.

HOW IS AYAHUASCA MADE?

Ayahuasca is typically made from the Banisteriopsis caapi vine and the leaves of the Psychotria viridis shrub.

The woody vine is cut into smaller pieces and pounded with a mallet into smaller fibers.

The leaves of the chacruna are gathered, washed, and combined with the macerated vine. Some brewers will alternate *b. caapi* and *p. viridis*, layering them over each other in the pot and then covering them with water. Together they are boiled for several hours, strained (the liquid is saved and set aside), and then the pot with plant material is filled with water and boiled again for several more hours. After straining this second batch, the plant material is put to one side, and all the liquid is combined and further boiled down slowly so as not to degrade the psychoactive ingredients.

Remember, ayahuasca is a Schedule 1 Controlled Substance. It is illegal to make your own ayahuasca in the U.S. and in most other countries because it contains the psychedelic DMT.

WILL YOU MAKE THE CHOICE TO TRY AYAHUASCA?

Over the years, it has been used by indigenous people for healing and spiritual purposes. In recent years, ayahuasca has gained popularity as a tool for treating various mental health conditions, including depression, anxiety, PTSD, and addiction. While there is some scientific evidence to support these claims, it is important to note that ayahuasca is a very powerful substance with potentially serious side effects. Therefore, it is critical to consult with a trained professional before drinking ayahuasca. While there are many reported benefits of ayahuasca, it is important to remember that it is a powerful psychedelic substance that should be treated with respect.

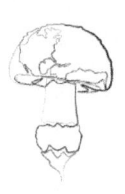

REFERENCES:

- Barbosa, P. C. R., Mizumoto, S., Bogenschutz, M. P., & Strassman, R. J. (2012). Health status of ayahuasca users. Drug Testing and Analysis, 4(7-8), 601-609. doi:https://doi.org/10.1002/dta.1383
- Callaway, J., & Grob, C. (1998). Ayahuasca Preparations and Serotonin Reuptake Inhibitors: A Potential Combination

for Severe Adverse Interactions. Journal of Psychoactive Drugs, 30, 367-369. doi:10.1080/02791072.1998.10399712
- Domínguez-Clavé, E., Soler, J., Elices, M., Pascual, J. C., Álvarez, E., de la Fuente Revenga, M., . . . Riba, J. (2016). Ayahuasca: Pharmacology, neuroscience and therapeutic potential. Brain Res Bull, 126(Pt 1), 89-101. doi:10.1016/j.brainresbull.2016.03.002
- Grob, C. S., & Grigsby, J. (2021). Handbook of Medical Hallucinogens: Guilford Publications.
- Guimarães dos Santos, R. (2013). Safety and Side Effects of Ayahuasca in Humans—An Overview Focusing on Developmental Toxicology. Journal of Psychoactive Drugs, 45(1), 68-78. doi:10.1080/02791072.2013.763564
- Hamill, J., Hallak, J., Dursun, S. M., & Baker, G. (2019). Ayahuasca: Psychological and Physiologic Effects, Pharmacology and Potential Uses in Addiction and Mental Illness. Curr Neuropharmacol, 17(2), 108-128. doi:10.2174/1570159x16666180125095902
- Palhano-Fontes, F., Barreto, D., Onias, H., Andrade, K. C., Novaes, M. M., Pessoa, J. A., . . . Araújo, D. B. (2019). Rapid antidepressant effects of the psychedelic ayahuasca in treatment-resistant depression: a randomized placebo-controlled trial. Psychological medicine, 49(4), 655-663. doi:10.1017/S0033291718001356

TWENTY-THREE
FINDING YOUR AYAHUASCA RETREAT
LEIA FRIEDWOMAN, MS

There is certainly something special about journeying to the ayahuasca plant's natural habitat to partake in a ceremony. The jungle is alive with energy, and it can be quite overwhelming if you're not used to being in such a lush, vibrant environment. If you're considering attending an ayahuasca retreat, it's important to do your research and choose a reputable center that feels right for you.

If you're considering flying down to Central or South America for an ayahuasca ceremony, here are some tips about how to choose the perfect retreat center, plus some thoughts on what to bring and what mental and physical preparation to do ahead of time.

HOW TO CHOOSE THE RIGHT RETREAT CENTER FOR YOU

When it comes to finding the right retreat center, the process can seem a bit daunting. There are so many different options available, and it can be hard to know where to start. By taking some time to understand what you're looking for, you can make the process much simpler.

When looking for a retreat center, do your research and make sure it's reputable. Search online for the name of the facility along with words like "scam" or "lawsuit," just in case there have been incidents there. The medicine facilitator(s) should be skilled and experienced in their work; many websites include a blurb about the lineage of their tradition. The staff should be well trained, professional, and appropriately equipped to deal with medical and psychological emergencies.

A reputable retreat center will screen participants extensively to ensure that ayahuasca is the right choice for them and that they are not likely to be a danger to themselves or others. Consider asking about the contents of the ayahuasca brew as well; some retreat centers have been known to include potentially dangerous plants in their recipes. Do your research to help ensure your safety and comfort.

Retreat centers vary based on location, accessibility, the lineage of the shaman, price, amenities, and reputation. Here are some considerations to keep in mind:

Choose a location that is accessible based on your travel needs and experience.

Ayahuasca is legal under cultural patrimony in Peru, meaning that the ceremonial and ritual use of the brew is regulated by the government. Colombia, Ecuador, and Costa Rica are also home to many retreat centers, although the governments of these countries do not regulate these centers.

Some centers, such as the Temple of the Way of Light in Peru, are not easily accessed. After flying in to Iquitos, the journey to the temple includes a motorbike ride, taxi or bus, big boat, small boat, and finally, a few miles walk down a muddy jungle path on foot. For some people, the beauty of the deep jungle, the level of isolation, and the adventure of the trek are desirable. Some will prefer a more accessible retreat center closer to a city or town, such as La Ceiba, outside of Medellin, Colombia.

When you go to a retreat center, make sure it has the amenities for your needs. For example, if you have specific medical or psychological needs, find a retreat with a medical facility close by.

Find a trained and reputable medicine person.

Some ayahuasca facilitators are indigenous, and some aren't. The training and integrity of the person leading your ceremony matter most; make sure to find someone who has significant experience serving the medicine. The facilitator should adopt clear physical boundaries; it is inappropriate for the shaman to engage with participants on intimate or sexual levels during the retreat at any time.

If sitting in ceremony with indigenous healers is important to you, there are plenty of retreats with amazing facilitators. Remember, some ayahuasca centers allow only minimal interaction with the shamans. However, you may be able to participate in intercultural activities such as medicine making, plant walks, and learning about tapestries and their significance.

Find a retreat that matches your budget.

There are retreats available for every budget. Whether you have a hundred Peruvian soles in your pocket or you're able to spend thousands on a deluxe retreat, you can find an establishment that works for you.

Some retreat centers come complete with swimming pools and spa options like massage, facials, reiki, reflexology, sound healing, and more. The accommodations at such a retreat may resemble a fancy hotel in terms of bedding, amenities, beauty, and comfort.

There are plenty of quality retreat centers with more affordable prices available. Sharing a tambo/room with another person is a way to cut down on costs. Just make sure that the center has all of your basic needs covered and that you'll be comfortable enough to be able to go deep into the ayahuasca experience.

Some retreats are more earthy and cater to nature lovers with their amenities. Staying in a rustic setting can be another way to "retreat" from the comforts of modern society and explore the sensations of a cold shower, a compost toilet, and candlelight.

No matter where you go, remember you are a guest in another country, so cultural practices may be different than you might expect in the U.S. or Europe. For example, nudity is commonly discouraged. Always be respectful and try to stay open to new ways of doing things; you may surprise yourself if you go outside of your comfort zone.

PRO-TIPS FOR TRAVELING TO THE JUNGLE TO DRINK AYAHUASCA

Make several copies of all your travel documents. It's good practice when traveling internationally to **make copies of your passport** and keep it in each piece of luggage. You should also email yourself a picture of your passport in case it gets lost.

Clearly and legibly **mark all of your luggage**, including contact information for how to reach you while you're abroad and back home. Have emergency contact information on you at all times.

Designate someone to take care of your personal affairs at home. Whether it's taking care of your pets, checking on your home, watering the plants, or something as serious as taking care of your child(ren), you should feel confident that your responsibilities are in the capable hands of a trusted person. There is enough to worry about already, and so the more you can delegate out your responsibilities, the more you can surrender to the experience.

Make sure you have enough money in the proper currency. Some countries in South and Central America, such as Costa Rica, will accept American money since they have such a large tourism industry. However, your bills must be clean, unmarked, unfolded, and relatively new. If you can acquire the foreign currency ahead of time, this may make things easier for you. You should be able to withdraw money from an ATM without much trouble, but make sure your PIN is four digits, as some foreign ATMs don't accept pins with more than four numbers.

Notify your bank and cell phone company that you'll be traveling internationally. Find out what your cell phone company offers for international trips. For a short stay, it may be more economical to go with their international plan (just make sure you follow their instructions so you don't end up racking up a huge unexpected cost). For longer trips, you can usually acquire a new sim card from a cellular provider in that country; sometimes, they even have them stationed at the airport. You typically need your passport in order to acquire a sim card.

But be cautious when using your cell phone while out in public. Stay focused on what you are doing and what's going on around you for safety reasons as well as to get the full benefit of this experience of visiting a new place. Looking at your phone is distracting and can be an invitation for someone to quickly swipe it out of your hands and disappear.

Learn some basic phrases in the native language of the country you're visiting. Even if you're insecure about your foreign language skills, locals will appreciate you trying to communicate in their tongue while you visit their home country. Plus, practice makes perfect, and what better opportunity to practice a new language than by challenging yourself to use it? Learn phrases such as:

- *Hello.*
- *Please. Thank you.*
- *Yes, No.*
- *Where is the bathroom?*
- *I don't speak_____.*
- *Do you speak English?*
- *I need help.*

Consider having a cheat sheet of common phrases easily accessible in your pocket or bag.

Be respectful and keep an open mind. Remember that you are a visitor to another country, so customs and norms can be different than what you are used to.

Learn about the culture before your trip. Try to stay open and humble while, of course, keeping yourself safe and having your boundaries. Respect local customs, such as refraining from nude swimming. Although there is nothing shameful about a naked body, nudity is considered inappropriate in many South and Central American cultures. Whether you agree with the custom or not, swimming nude is an act of colonialism. Following these customs is a sign of respect and gratitude for being able to visit someone else's home.

Just as psychedelic work is a balance of effort and surrender, packing for your ayahuasca retreat is a balance of being prepared and not overpacking. Don't leave home without these ten items.

MUST-HAVE ITEMS FOR A TRIP TO THE JUNGLE

1. A really good water bottle. Travel can be dehydrating, especially in a hot climate. Staying hydrated before your ayahuasca experience is very important. On travel days, try to balance hydration with practicality; you don't want to have to use the bathroom at every stop if you can avoid it. Remember, bottled water is safer than tap water in foreign countries. There are many UV light and portable filtration devices for travelers to purify their water as well.

2. Non-toxic sun protection and insect repellent.
Sunglasses or a hat will come in handy. Non-toxic insect repellents are safer to use and help protect you as well as the flora and fauna around you from harmful chemicals like DEET. If you're concerned about insect-borne disease, wearing long-sleeved clothing and spraying on natural insecticides should protect you well enough. Outdoor equipment retailers sell mosquito-proof suits that may be worth the price for your protection and peace of mind.

3. Eco-friendly travel toiletries. Most ayahuasca retreat centers are in nature, so bringing biodegradable, natural products is greatly appreciated in order to not contaminate the natural environment. Dr. Bronner's soap is a versatile option as it can be used to wash dishes and clothing as well as your hair and body. It's concentrated, so you can bring a small amount, dilute it on arrival and have it last your whole trip.

4. Headlamp or flashlight. Most ayahuasca ceremonies take place at night. The jungle is crawling with thousands of amazing creatures; shine your light so you can make sure not to step on them (and avoid potentially hurting yourself). A headlamp with multiple light settings, especially red light, will help you get to the bathroom during the ceremony without disturbing the other participants.

5. Prescription and non-prescription medications. Talk to your doctor before your trip about what medication to bring with you. Some doctors will prescribe an antibiotic that you can have with you just in case you need it and can't access a pharmacy. Find out if there is malaria in the region you're visiting and if there is, ask about anti-malaria medication (and make sure it is safe to combine with Ayahuasca). You could look into herbal options such as Artemesia. Remember to let the ayahuasca retreat center know about any medications, and do not take anything that is contraindicated with ayahuasca. Find out if certain vaccinations are required or recommended for the country you are visiting, and take care of those ahead of time.

6. The right clothing. Pack plenty of layers. Quick-drying, breathable fabrics are best for tropical climates. Temperatures can drop at night, and you could become very cold or shivery during the ceremony, so have at least one good set of warm clothes. A bathing suit, travel towel, clothes for walking or hiking outside, clothes for yoga, and clothes for travel days are all smart to have:

> a. Bring enough underwear to last a week, just in case. Underwear made for travel is quick-drying, lightweight, and antimicrobial. You can always wash and dry it in your room if laundry services are unavailable.

> b. The humidity in the jungle lends itself to mold, so don't bring anything with you that you wouldn't want to get mold

stained. Moving clothing, shoes, and bags to a new spot in your room every day can help stop the spread of mold. c. Hanging things out in the sun daily is another great trick.

c. Sarongs are a wonderful travel option as they can be used as clothing, a light blanket to cover yourself with or sit on outside, a makeshift towel to dry off with, sun protection in a pinch, and more.

d. Touristy places will have plenty of clothing you can buy in case you don't have something that you need.

7. Comfortable shoes. A pair of shoes that are easy to put on/take off, such as flip-flops, will come in handy. If it's the rainy season, consider bringing rain boots. If they are in good condition, you can always leave them behind for someone else to use, so you don't have to bring them home with you. It's wise to bring shoes that you can walk comfortably in for long distances. If you plan to hike, make sure you are equipped for that. New shoes are a risky idea; whatever you bring should be broken in, so you avoid getting blisters.

8. Hair ties or bandana. Motorbike and bus rides can get windy. Make sure you have what you need to keep your hair in place. In ceremony, it's advised to have something that holds your hair back while you are purging.

9. Journal. Bring paper, a pen/pencil, and even some portable art supplies with you to record thoughts and visions from your ayahuasca experience in the hours and days following the ceremony. Drawing, coloring, writing down dreams, and freewriting are all great activities to capture the musings that arise while you are on retreat. And, since many retreat centers have no Wi-Fi or very limited WIFI, it could be good to have something to spend time on. A book or two can also be great to bring with you as a way to relax during the daytime.

10. Plastic or Waterproof Bags. There is nothing quite like a sudden rainstorm in the jungle. One minute it can be clear blue skies, and the next you are hustling to save your stuff from the buckets of water falling from above. Keep plastic bags such as big trash bags in the exterior pockets of your luggage and backpack so you can easily take them out and cover everything. Small waterproof bags are great for protecting electronics and wallets.

WHAT NOT TO BRING

A list of what to bring is not complete without a list of what not to bring. Consider leaving the following items behind:

- valuable jewelry.
- too much cash.
- technological devices, other than your cell phone (Consider just bringing the bare minimum when it comes to technology, so you don't have to devote energy to worrying about it being lost, stolen, or damaged. The rainforest is humid and could wreak havoc on your devices if not stored properly. Most importantly, a retreat is an opportunity to unplug and get in touch with yourself. Taking a break from tech may be powerful medicine.)
- unnecessary items that will weigh you down, like lots of books.
- makeup; no one will be worried about whether or not you're wearing mascara.

Anything else you think you "might" need…you probably won't.

PART SIX
MDMA

"It [MDMA] takes away the feelings of self-hatred and condemnation, which are the biggest obstacles to insight… For reasons we don't understand, MDMA allows people to do this, typically in one [psychotherapeutic] session."

Ann Shulgin

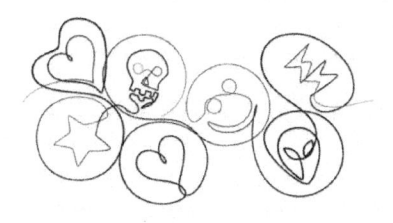

TWENTY-FOUR
A BEGINNER'S GUIDE TO MDMA
AMELIA WALSH

MEDICALLY REVIEWED BY DR. LYNN-MARIE MORSKI, MD, JD

Although it has a reputation as a party drug, for many, the appeal of MDMA lies in its potential to be used as a catalyst for psychotherapy and exploration. It garners the attention of both supporters and skeptics because of its potential for both therapeutic support and for misuse.

Brother David Steindl-Rast told the *Los Angeles Times* the MDMA experience was "like climbing all day in the fog and then suddenly, briefly seeing the mountain peak for the first time. There are no shortcuts to the awakened attitude, and it takes daily work and effort. But the drug gives you a vision, a glimpse of what you are seeking."

Understanding MDMA and its effects will help clarify uncertainties about the potential benefits and risks.

AN OVERVIEW OF MDMA

4-Methylenedioxy-methamphetamine (MDMA) is a synthetic, psychoactive substance best known for producing a euphoric state with simultaneous stimulant and psychedelic effects. MDMA was first synthesized in 1912 by German chemists and was eventually patented by the drug company Merck. It was briefly used by the CIA during the Cold War as part of Project MK-Ultra, a program to explore the potential use of psychedelics for mind control. MDMA was resynthesized in 1965 by Alexander "Sasha" Shulgin. In the mid-1970's Shulgin introduced MDMA to Leo Zeff, PhD, who began using it along with psychotherapy and introducing it to other psychotherapists.

Friederike Meckel Fisher and other practitioners of psychedelic-assisted psychotherapy advocated for MDMA's use as a tool in both individual sessions and couples counseling, saying it "alleviates fear" and enables people to "access parts of their minds they might normally suppress" (Trope et al., 2019).

The Nixon administration enacted the Controlled Substances Act in 1970, declaring a 'War on Drugs." MDMA was listed as a Schedule 1 drug and became banned in 1985 after it had become popular among recreational users.

The change in legal status did little to alter the popularity of MDMA as the main ingredient of drugs used in social settings such as electronic dance music (EDM) or 'rave' events, though when produced outside of clinical settings, it is often found to be contaminated with a variety of other substances. In recreational use, MDMA is also commonly referred to as ecstasy, molly, or E.

It continues to be the subject of research, with growing evidence for the benefits of MDMA-assisted therapy in treating post-traumatic stress disorder (PTSD) and social anxiety in adults with autism. The U.S. Food and Drug Administration (FDA) recently awarded Breakthrough Therapy designation to MDMA-assisted psychotherapy for PTSD, which expedites the processing of study findings and allows the potential for a quicker path to approval for therapeutic use (Feduccia & Mithoefer, 2018).

HOW MDMA WORKS

The effects of MDMA are produced by increasing levels of hormones and the neurotransmitters serotonin (5-HT), dopamine (DA), and norepinephrine (N.E.) (de la Torre et al., 2004). Serotonin is partially responsible for mood regulation. MDMA triggers the release of serotonin and simultaneously blocks its reuptake temporarily, allowing for buildup in the brain. Dopamine affects the reward processing function of the brain, making interactions feel more meaningful and boosting energy. Increased norepinephrine levels cause elevated blood pressure and heart rate.

METHODS OF INTAKE

MDMA can be ingested orally in the form of tablets, capsules, or powder. It is also possible to snort and absorb it through the nose by way of mucous membranes, which allows for quicker effects. As of now, information is lacking on the prevalence, effects, and risks of smoking or injecting MDMA, as these methods are far less common.

IS MDMA THE SAME AS MOLLY OR ECSTASY?

MDMA is the scientific term, but recreational users often refer to MDMA as molly or ecstasy. Assumption of its purity is common; however, MDMA which hasn't been formulated by research scientists is commonly adulterated with other substances in recreational forms of the drug. Street drugs that claim to be MDMA may have little to no MDMA content.

MDMA EFFECTS AND BENEFITS

The characteristic positive effect of MDMA is euphoria. Depending on one's mindset, companions, and environment, it can manifest in a variety of ways. Feelings of connectedness to the inner self and other people, a heightened sense of spirituality, being more social or open to new ideas and experiences, increased arousal and awareness of physical sensations, meaningful interaction with art and music, mild visual and auditory hallucinations, and generally feeling at peace are a few examples.

While these effects make MDMA a popular recreational enhancement for creative and social events, as evidenced by the research cited above, many have reported transformative, intimate experiences through taking the drug in more formal, therapeutic settings.

HOW LONG DOES MDMA LAST?

Depending on several factors, the effects of MDMA can last anywhere from 3 to 6 hours after a single dose of unadulterated MDMA (Sessa, 2017). Re-dosing might extend the length of efficacy for a certain amount of time depending on tolerance and medications, other substances, or health considerations.

A study of urine samples taken from a group of participants given a single oral dose of MDMA showed that most of the substance was excreted through urine within the first 24 hours after application (Abraham et al., 2009). Depending on the individual, dosage, testing method, and scope, MDMA has been detected in trial participants within the first hour of oral intake and up to 7 days later (Abraham et al., 2009).

RESEARCH AND CURRENT USES

In the 1960s and '70s, MDMA became a tool for lowering the inhibitions people often feel when reflecting on painful and traumatic experiences, allegedly resulting in more productive therapy sessions, according to the few therapists who utilized it (Passie, 2018). Although it was banned as a recreational drug in 1985, MDMA has shown promise in clinical studies of the benefits demonstrated when treating severe post-traumatic stress disorder (PTSD) in cases where conventional methods alone have been insufficient (Mithoefer et al., 2013). It was approved for Breakthrough Therapy designation by the U.S. Food and Drug Administration (FDA) in 2017, allowing expedited development and review of a substance that shows promise in treating serious conditions.

Such a designation also requires proposed drugs to demonstrate the likelihood of "substantial improvement over available therapies" in existing studies. It is now in phase 3 trials for the treatment of PTSD, with a specific protocol for MDMA-assisted therapy studies sponsored and outlined by The Multidisciplinary Association for Psychedelic Studies (MAPS).

Research has also focused on MDMA as a possible treatment for severe social anxiety in adults with autism when conventional approaches failed to improve symptoms (Danforth, Struble, Yazar-Klosinski, & Grob, 2016). There was encouraging, conclusive data showing improvements in the LSAS (Leibowitz Social Anxiety Scale) score for the group administered MDMA, described in the study results as 'significantly greater' than the recipients of placebo.

Very recently, researchers have begun to explore whether MDMA-assisted psychotherapy could possibly be effective in the treatment of eating disorders (Brewerton, Lafrance, & Mithoefer, 2021)and anxiety in adults coping with a life-threatening illness (Wolfson et al., 2020).

People in relationships have also leveraged the feelings of connectedness facilitated by MDMA in the context of therapy, particularly when one or both suffer from PTSD or the effects of trauma that can impact the dynamic of a partnership.

The impact of MDMA in the treatment of PTSD is dependent on its use in conjunction with psychotherapy. MDMA appears to help dismantle some of the emotional defense mechanisms that hinder survivors of trauma from benefiting from a psychotherapeutic session, such as a tendency to withdraw or become overwhelmed and upset when the therapeutic session becomes challenging. Research also suggests that it might minimize reactions of distress in discussions that would otherwise trigger a negative emotional response.

Research speculates that MDMA can facilitate trust with a therapist that is otherwise established over years of difficult effort, if at all (Mithoefer et al., 2013). This is likely because, in addition to promoting the release of several monoamine transmitters (primarily serotonin or 5-HT) and temporarily preventing their reuptake, it increases levels of serum oxytocin. This neuropeptide is thought to be partially responsible for bonding in mammals. As Anne Wagner (Adjunct Professor of Psychology at Ryerson University) describes it, MDMA-assisted psychotherapy offers the hope "to move the seemingly immovable presence of the trauma."

MDMA SIDE EFFECTS AND RISKS

Side effects of MDMA are common and range from mild to severe (Droogmans et al., 2007). Clenching teeth, elevated body temperature with the risk of hyperthermia, dry mouth, sweating, hyponatremia, nausea, diarrhea, muscle cramps, blurry vision, reduced appetite, tremors, and chills are some of the possible adverse physical effects (Steinkellner, Freissmuth, Sitte, &

Montgomery, 2011). When heart rate and blood pressure increase after the administration of MDMA, there is a risk of serious complications for those with existing heart disease and other health issues. MDMA also has the potential to interact poorly with prescription medications or in combination with different substances.

The acute psychological side effects most often reported are anxiety and paranoia, sometimes with visual or auditory hallucinations. Long-term effects of MDMA abuse include depression, problems with memory and attention, and damage to the brain's serotonin neurons. You may also be at risk for developing psychotic symptoms such as paranoia and delusions if you have a history of mental illness.

Cases of fatal overdose from MDMA alone are rare considering its underground popularity, but polydrug use and the related deaths are not accounted for in data examining exclusive usage of MDMA. In the days following the use of MDMA, symptoms like depression and fatigue are likely due to depleted levels of serotonin and exhaustion following recreational use on weekends.

Increasingly frequent use of MDMA can lead to the development of tolerance and, therefore, dependency, requiring increased dosage to experience the effects.

IS MDMA SAFE?

Psychoactive substances like MDMA have both psychological and physical effects that can be unsafe for a variety of reasons. A study with acute administration demonstrated that MDMA appears to be safe for healthy adults with benefits outweighing adverse effects, but it also noted the risks for those with health concerns or diagnoses of cardiovascular and psychiatric disorders (Vizeli & Liechti, 2017).

Outside of a professional therapeutic setting, there is significant concern about substance purity. Tablets, crystals, and powders sold illegally and called molly or ecstasy have been found to be up to 90 percent impure, containing 18 different substances across 1,232 samples in a probe of substances seized by police (Murray et al., 2003). Contaminants like synthetic stimulants and new psychoactive substances are undetectable without testing.

While test kits are commercially available, an analysis of the accuracy in reagent test kit results revealed a lack of test accuracy. More accurate and accessible testing methods are required in order to effectively facilitate harm reduction.

Hair samples of users who self-reported the use of MDMA, molly, or ecstasy within a year of the study revealed that 51.1 percent of participants tested positive for substances they didn't report. Seventy-two percent tested positive for synthetic cathinones, which are stimulant drugs known more commonly as 'bath salts.' Methamphetamine and speed (amphetamine) were found in 49.2 percent of samples containing a substance other than MDMA in a survey of participants who used a test kit to determine the purity of a substance they intended to take.

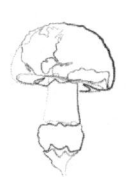

REFERENCES:

- Abraham, T. T., Barnes, A. J., Lowe, R. H., Kolbrich Spargo, E. A., Milman, G., Pirnay, S. O., . . . Huestis, M. A. (2009). Urinary MDMA, MDA, HMMA, and HMA excretion following controlled MDMA administration to humans. *Journal of analytical toxicology, 33*(8), 439-446. doi:10.1093/jat/33.8.439

- Brewerton, T. D., Lafrance, A., & Mithoefer, M. C. (2021). The potential use of N-methyl-3,4-methylenedioxyamphetamine (MDMA) assisted psychotherapy in the treatment of eating disorders comorbid with PTSD. *Med Hypotheses, 146*, 110367. doi:10.1016/j.mehy.2020.110367
- Danforth, A. L., Struble, C. M., Yazar-Klosinski, B., & Grob, C. S. (2016). MDMA-assisted therapy: A new treatment model for social anxiety in autistic adults. *Prog Neuropsychopharmacol Biol Psychiatry, 64*, 237-249. doi:10.1016/j.pnpbp.2015.03.011
- de la Torre, R., Farré, M., Roset, P. N., Pizarro, N., Abanades, S., Segura, M., . . . Camí, J. (2004). Human Pharmacology of MDMA: Pharmacokinetics, Metabolism, and Disposition. *Therapeutic Drug Monitoring, 26*(2), 137-144. Retrieved from https://journals.lww.com/drug-monitoring/Fulltext/2004/04000/Human_Pharmacology_of_MDMA__Pharmacokinetics,.9.aspx
- Droogmans, S., Cosyns, B., D'Haenen, H., Creeten, E., Weytjens, C., Franken, P. R., . . . Van Camp, G. (2007). Possible association between 3,4-methylenedioxymethamphetamine abuse and valvular heart disease. *Am J Cardiol, 100*(9), 1442-1445. doi:10.1016/j.amjcard.2007.06.045
- Feduccia, A. A., & Mithoefer, M. C. (2018). MDMA-assisted psychotherapy for PTSD: Are memory reconsolidation and fear extinction underlying mechanisms? *Prog Neuropsychopharmacol Biol Psychiatry, 84*(Pt A), 221-228. doi:10.1016/j.pnpbp.2018.03.003
- Mithoefer, M. C., Wagner, M. T., Mithoefer, A. T., Jerome, L., Martin, S. F., Yazar-Klosinski, B., . . . Doblin, R. (2013). Durability of improvement in post-traumatic stress disorder symptoms and absence of harmful effects or drug dependency after 3,4-methylenedioxymethamphetamine-

- assisted psychotherapy: a prospective long-term follow-up study. *Journal of psychopharmacology (Oxford, England), 27*(1), 28-39. doi:10.1177/0269881112456611
- Murray, R. A., Doering, P. L., Boothby, L. A., Merves, M. L., McCusker, R. R., Chronister, C. W., & Goldberger, B. A. (2003). Putting an Ecstasy test kit to the test: harm reduction or harm induction? *Pharmacotherapy, 23*(10), 1238-1244. doi:10.1592/phco.23.12.1238.32704
- Passie, T. (2018). The early use of MDMA ('Ecstasy') in psychotherapy (1977–1985). *Drug Science, Policy and Law, 4*, 2050324518767442. doi:10.1177/2050324518767442
- Sessa, B. (2017). MDMA and PTSD treatment: "PTSD: From novel pathophysiology to innovative therapeutics". *Neuroscience Letters, 649*, 176-180. doi:https://doi.org/10.1016/j.neulet.2016.07.004
- Steinkellner, T., Freissmuth, M., Sitte, H. H., & Montgomery, T. (2011). The ugly side of amphetamines: short- and long-term toxicity of 3,4-methylenedioxymethamphetamine (MDMA, 'Ecstasy'), methamphetamine and D-amphetamine. *Biological chemistry, 392*(1-2), 103-115. doi:10.1515/BC.2011.016
- Trope, A., Anderson, B. T., Hooker, A. R., Glick, G., Stauffer, C., & Woolley, J. D. (2019). Psychedelic-Assisted Group Therapy: A Systematic Review. *Journal of Psychoactive Drugs, 51*(2), 174-188. doi:10.1080/02791072.2019.1593559
- Vizeli, P., & Liechti, M. E. (2017). Safety pharmacology of acute MDMA administration in healthy subjects. *Journal of psychopharmacology (Oxford, England), 31*(5), 576-588. doi:10.1177/0269881117691569
- Wolfson, P. E., Andries, J., Feduccia, A. A., Jerome, L., Wang, J. B., Williams, E., . . . Doblin, R. (2020). MDMA-assisted psychotherapy for treatment of anxiety and other psychological distress related to life-threatening illnesses: a

randomized pilot study. *Scientific Reports, 10*(1), 20442. doi:10.1038/s41598-020-75706-1

TWENTY-FIVE
MDMA AND PTSD
AMBER KRAUS

MEDICALLY REVIEWED BY DR. LYNN-MARIE MORSKI, MD, JD

After a traumatic event, it is not uncommon for people to feel scared, confused, or sad. For most people, these symptoms will fade over time as they come to terms with what happened. However, for some people, these feelings do not go away and can even get worse. This is known as post-traumatic stress disorder (PTSD). People with PTSD may re-experience the trauma through nightmares and flashbacks, may avoid people and places associated with the trauma, and might feel emotionally numb.

Some research suggests that combining MDMA with psychotherapy may help patients to process their traumas more effectively without feeling overwhelmed or flooded with anxiety. In addition, the positive mood induced by MDMA may help to create a more trusting environment in which patients can feel safe enough to explore their memories and emotions. While further research is needed to confirm the efficacy of this treatment approach, the preliminary results are promising and offer hope for those who suffer from this debilitating condition.

In December 2019, the FDA approved the Multidisciplinary Association for Psychedelic Studies (MAPS) for an expanded access program of MDMA-assisted psychotherapy for the treatment of PTSD (Feduccia et al., 2019). While the therapeutic protocol is still being tested, this program will allow for "early access to potentially beneficial investigational therapies for people facing a serious or life-threatening condition for whom currently available treatments have not worked, and who are unable to participate in Phase 3 clinical trials."

PTSD SYMPTOMS

Post-Traumatic Stress Disorder (PTSD) is a complex condition that can develop in response to any number of traumatic events. While the symptoms of PTSD can vary widely in severity, they all share one common trait: they serve to remind the sufferer of the trauma they have experienced. For many people, this can lead to a downward spiral of avoidance behavior, insomnia, and negative self-talk. They may constantly be on guard for danger, have difficulty sleeping, or be easily startled. They may also have trouble concentrating or remembering key features of the trauma. In some cases, people with PTSD may have outbursts toward people who are perceived to be like those associated with the original trauma.

Complex post-traumatic stress disorder (C-PTSD) occurs when a person has been exposed to multiple types of trauma over an extended period of time. This can include situations such as chronic childhood abuse or domestic violence. C-PTSD is often more severe and longer-lasting than regular post-traumatic stress disorder (PTSD), as the individual continues to be exposed to the traumatic situation on a recurring basis.

COMPLEX PTSD SYMPTOMS CAN INCLUDE:

1. Behavior difficulties. People who have experienced prolonged or repeated exposure to traumatic events may struggle with aggressiveness and impulsivity. They may misuse drugs or alcohol or participate in self-destructive behavior.

2. Emotional difficulties. Those who experience PTSD can struggle with regulating their emotions and may experience strong emotional reactions triggered by certain events. They may experience outbursts of anger or rage and an inability to control their responses to stressful situations. Many people who suffer from PTSD struggle to cope with the everyday stressors of life effectively.

3. Cognitive difficulties. PTSD can alter cognitive processes such as attention, problem-solving, planning, and memory. This can make it difficult to concentrate at work or to complete everyday tasks or routines.

4. Interpersonal difficulties. Feelings of isolation or loneliness are common in people who have experienced PTSD. Survivors of PTSD often feel little emotional connection with others and may feel that their experiences have made them different from others or that they are psychologically damaged or broken and unable to create bonds and connections with others.

5. Somatization. Somatization occurs when psychological concerns manifest as physical symptoms such as pain, weakness, or shortness of breath. They may experience other physical symptoms, such as chronic fatigue or gastrointestinal issues.

According to research by Michael Mithoefer, MD, in the United States Military the incidence of PTSD in people returning from [the war in] Iraq was as high as 18%, and in fact, more soldiers returning from Iraq and Afghanistan have committed suicide from untreated PTSD than actually died in the conflict. (Michael C. Mithoefer et al., 2013).

MDMA AS AN ADJUNCT TO PSYCHOTHERAPY

MDMA (3,4-methylenedioxymethamphetamine) is a synthetic drug that was originally developed as an adjunct to psychotherapy. In the 1980s, MDMA became increasingly popular as a "party drug," and it remains one of the most commonly used recreational drugs today. Despite its popularity as a party drug, MDMA's therapeutic applications have been studied and endorsed by medical professionals for decades. MDMA has been shown to be an effective treatment for a variety of conditions, including post-traumatic stress disorder (PTSD), anxiety, and depression. It is also being studied as a potential treatment for substance abuse disorders. While MDMA is not currently approved by the FDA for any therapeutic use, its therapeutic potential is widely recognized by medical professionals.

The recent success of MDMA-assisted psychotherapy in clinical trials offers hope for those who suffer from PTSD and have not seen success with more conventional treatment programs. In fact, in a study of subjects with treatment-resistant PTSD, 56% of patients who received MDMA-assisted therapy no longer met DSM-IV criteria for PTSD immediately following the study (Jerome et al., 2020). Patients reported that their PTSD symptoms improved for at least a year after the experience. Follow-up studies indicated that 67% of those whose PTSD symptoms improved no longer met the clinical qualifications for a diagnosis of PTSD at the twelve-month mark after study completion (Mitchell et al., 2021).

In 2017 the FDA granted Breakthrough Therapy Designation for MDMA -assisted psychotherapy in the treatment of PTSD. Breakthrough Therapy Designation is "a process designed to expedite the development and review of drugs that are intended to treat a serious condition and preliminary clinical evidence indicates that the drug may demonstrate substantial improvement over available therapy on a clinically significant endpoint(s)."

Phase III studies on MDMA for PTSD are still in the early stages, but continued research will further explore how MDMA-assisted therapy can help heal the psychological and emotional damage caused by sexual assault, war, violent crime, and other traumas (M. C. Mithoefer et al., 2019).

MDMA, ECSTASY, AND MOLLY: ARE THEY ALL THE SAME?

When people think of MDMA, they often think of the party drug known as ecstasy or molly. However, the MDMA that is being discussed here is not necessarily the same as what is found in those drugs. These substances often contain unknown and dangerous adulterants (Palamar, 2017), which can be harmful to users. In laboratory studies, pure MDMA has been proven sufficiently safe for human consumption when taken in limited quantities on occasion with moderate doses (Feduccia et al., 2019; Jerome et al., 2020; Wolfson et al., 2020).

Since MDMA is currently unregulated, anything sold as "molly" or "ecstasy" could range from pure MDMA to MDMA mixed with other drugs to containing no MDMA at all. The molly market is one of the most adulterated illicit drug markets, meaning it often is cut with other substances.

This is in stark contrast to the MDMA used in FDA-approved clinical studies for the treatment of PTSD. In PTSD therapy it is used in a regulated setting, usually on two occasions over the course of several weeks, and alongside talk therapy with one or more therapists.

BENEFITS OF MDMA FOR PTSD

MDMA is not known to cause any serious side effects when taken in appropriate quantities and in a controlled setting. Studies have shown that MDMA therapy can be safe and effective when accompanied by psychotherapy (Mitchell et al., 2021). The unique effect of MDMA in reducing fear and enhancing interpersonal trust makes it especially helpful for healing psychological damage from traumas. Because fear and loss of trust are the basis for many symptoms of PTSD, MDMA has great potential for curing PTSD by working with the brain and mind to help people overcome fear.

MDMA can help provide relief from symptoms of PTSD in those suffering from this condition by making people more sympathetic to one another, and the drug has been known to decrease feelings of anger and hostility (Mitchell et al., 2021).

In short, the use of MDMA as an adjunct to psychotherapy for PTSD treatment can produce long-lasting improvements in the symptoms of PTSD.

HOW DOES MDMA HELP THOSE WITH PTSD?

Several studies have shown that MDMA reduces activity in the emotional centers of the brain, including the amygdala and hippocampus (Morey et al., 2012). This may be responsible for how it helps patients overcome their painful memories. The amygdala and hippocampus work together to process emotions. Because people who experience PTSD exhibit hyperactivity in the amygdala, they may experience emotions in a more extreme and unregulated way than they did before the trauma. With the use of MDMA, there is decreased activity in those areas of the brain, thus reducing the extremity of emotional responses and allowing for deeper processing of the traumatic event.

CAN PTSD BE CURED?

In recent years, scientists have made significant progress in understanding and treating PTSD. Although there is currently no cure for the condition, a combination of medication and therapy can effectively minimize symptoms such as flashbacks, insomnia, anxiety, and depression.

The most common medications used to treat PTSD are selective serotonin reuptake inhibitors (SSRIs), which are antidepressants that help to regulate levels of the neurotransmitter serotonin. Therapies such as exposure therapy and cognitive-behavioral therapy (CBT) have also been shown to be effective in reducing symptoms.

The synthetic psychoactive chemical MDMA is emerging as a promising treatment for PTSD. Research has shown significant improvement in those treated with MDMA's therapeutic properties rather than traditional treatments, which have proven less effective in the past.

There is no one-size-fits-all approach to treating PTSD. Some individuals respond better to a specific treatment than others. Self-management strategies such as mindfulness and meditation work for some people, and alternative treatments like psychotherapy and having a service dog work for others.

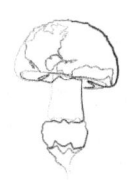

REFERENCES:

- Feduccia, A. A., Jerome, L., Yazar-Klosinski, B., Emerson, A., Mithoefer, M. C., & Doblin, R. (2019). Breakthrough for Trauma Treatment: Safety and Efficacy of MDMA-Assisted Psychotherapy Compared to Paroxetine and Sertraline. *Front Psychiatry, 10*, 650. doi:10.3389/fpsyt.2019.00650
- Jerome, L., Feduccia, A. A., Wang, J. B., Hamilton, S., Yazar-Klosinski, B., Emerson, A., . . . Doblin, R. (2020). Long-term follow-up outcomes of MDMA-assisted psychotherapy for treatment of PTSD: a longitudinal pooled analysis of six phase 2 trials. *Psychopharmacology, 237*(8), 2485-2497. doi:10.1007/s00213-020-05548-2
- Mitchell, J. M., Bogenschutz, M., Lilienstein, A., Harrison, C., Kleiman, S., Parker-Guilbert, K., . . . Doblin, R. (2021). MDMA-assisted therapy for severe PTSD: a randomized, double-blind, placebo-controlled phase 3 study. *Nature Medicine, 27*(6), 1025-1033. doi:10.1038/s41591-021-01336-3
- Mithoefer, M. C., Feduccia, A. A., Jerome, L., Mithoefer, A., Wagner, M., Walsh, Z., . . . Doblin, R. (2019). MDMA-assisted psychotherapy for treatment of PTSD: study design and rationale for phase 3 trials based on pooled analysis of six phase 2 randomized controlled trials. *Psychopharmacology (Berl), 236*(9), 2735-2745. doi:10.1007/s00213-019-05249-5

- Mithoefer, M. C., Wagner, M. T., Mithoefer, A. T., Jerome, L., Martin, S. F., Yazar-Klosinski, B., . . . Doblin, R. (2013). Durability of improvement in post-traumatic stress disorder symptoms and absence of harmful effects or drug dependency after 3,4-methylenedioxymethamphetamine-assisted psychotherapy: a prospective long-term follow-up study. *Journal of psychopharmacology (Oxford, England), 27*(1), 28-39. doi:10.1177/0269881112456611
- Morey, R. A., Gold, A. L., LaBar, K. S., Beall, S. K., Brown, V. M., Haswell, C. C., . . . Mid-Atlantic, M. W. (2012). Amygdala volume changes in posttraumatic stress disorder in a large case-controlled veterans group. *Archives of General Psychiatry, 69*(11), 1169-1178. doi:10.1001/archgenpsychiatry.2012.50

PART SEVEN
LSD

"These tools make it possible to study important processes that under normal circumstances are not available for direct observation."

Dr. Stanislav Grof, MD

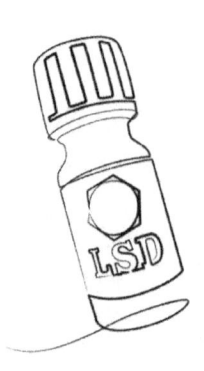

TWENTY-SIX
A BEGINNER'S GUIDE TO LSD
AMBER KRAUS

MEDICALLY REVIEWED BY DR. DAVID COX, PHD, ABPP

Lysergic acid diethylamide (LSD) is a powerful psychoactive substance that was first synthesized in 1938 by Swiss chemist Albert Hofmann. LSD's impacts on human consciousness were first discovered on April 19th, 1943, when Hofmann intentionally ingested the substance to ascertain its effects (an event which later came to be known as Bicycle Day). LSD produces profound changes in perception, thought, and emotion that can last 12 hours or longer. The exact mechanism by which LSD produces these changes is not fully understood, though it is believed to involve disruptions to serotonin signaling in the brain.

The main ingredient in LSD is lysergic acid, which is derived from ergot, a type of fungus that grows on rye and other grains. Ergot has been used medicinally for centuries; in the 1500s, midwives began using it to help ease labor pains. In the 20th century, LSD was first used recreationally before becoming known for its therapeutic benefits. Today, clinical research has shown that LSD can be an effective treatment for alcohol and opiate addictions. (Dyck, 2006; Krebs & Johansen, 2012).

Many people are apprehensive about taking LSD because of the cultural baggage surrounding its use. During the 1960s counterculture movement, LSD became popularized through the likes of Timothy Leary, an ex-Harvard psychologist who publicly encouraged young Americans to "turn on, tune in, drop out." Rising in popularity amongst America's youth, LSD quickly gained a reputation as a party drug. Adding to this, its use was demonized by the Nixon administration, who declared Timothy Leary "the most dangerous man in America" and formally declared the "War on Drugs."

However, as scientific research into psychedelics continues to grow, it has been shown that LSD can help people have meaningful experiences, giving way to insightful new ideas (Schmid, Gasser, Oehen, & Liechti, 2020; Schmid & Liechti, 2018). To some extent, the effects of LSD can be unpredictable, but the most common ones include altered and/or enhanced sensory perception and changes in thought patterns.

People who are under the influence of LSD may experience visual and other sensory distortions, changes to their thought processes, as well as intense emotions such as euphoria. People have reported experiencing surprising or new insights while on the drug.

Research has identified a neural system, the Default Mode Network (DMN), which is typically activated when a person is daydreaming or otherwise engaged in non-directive thought or tasks. It is believed that LSD and other psychedelics may interact with the DMN in producing the effects that occur while on the substance (Nichols, 2016; Smigielski, Scheidegger, Kometer, & Vollenweider, 2019).

FORMS OF LSD

There are over 100 types of LSD on the market today, and they fall into four main categories: blotter paper, liquid solutions, tablets/microdots, and gelatin sheets. LSD on blotter paper is the most common form of the substance.

Blotter Paper

LSD blotter is typically divided into about 1/4" squares, referred to as "tabs." The dose in a single tab may vary, yet the full experience of LSD can be expected somewhere between 100μg-200μg of LSD (Liechti, 2017). It is often suggested that a lower dose be taken when using LSD for the first time. Paper blotters are created by taking a sheet of absorbent paper and soaking it in a liquid dilution of LSD. The dosage can vary greatly from one batch to another. Because of the method used to make blotter tabs, there is no practical way to know the exact dosage of a particular tab without either testing it or knowing the chemist. Adjacent tabs on a sheet will usually contain very similar levels of LSD.

Liquid LSD

LSD is water-soluble and is usually dissolved in alcohol or water. There are two main methods of taking liquid LSD. One way is to add it to a beverage and drink it. The second method, which requires more caution but produces a stronger effect on the body more quickly, is to place drops of the liquid underneath the tongue. A single drop of liquid LSD could be very strong, so it's important to measure your dose to avoid ingesting too much and to minimize undesirable effects.

Gelatin or Sugar Cubes

LSD in gelatin form is also known as "windowpanes." It is made by mixing liquid LSD with gelatin and forming it into small, thin squares. Similarly, liquid LSD can be mixed into sugar cubes.

SAFETY FIRST

When deciding on whether to take LSD or not, safety should be the number one priority. No matter the purpose for or method of taking LSD, one should take note of the following safety precautions:

1. **Avoid taking LSD if you are pregnant or have certain health conditions.** If someone chooses to take LSD, they should be in generally good health. If there is a personal or family history of schizophrenia, bipolar disorder, or other psychotic disorders, LSD and other psychedelics should be avoided.
2. **Avoid taking LSD when taking medications that it may interact adversely with.** One should avoid the use of LSD while taking tricyclic antidepressants or lithium. Mixing LSD with MDMA or cannabis may increase the chances of having a challenging trip because it can increase the hallucinogenic effects, although some people choose to mix LSD with MDMA or cannabis to experience a different trip and, in the case of cannabis, perhaps reduce nausea (Schechter, 1998).
3. **Test your LSD.** It is important to be 100% sure that what is being ingested is pure LSD. LSD and other psychedelic drugs, when purchased from non-reputable sources, can sometimes be mixed with other dangerous substances. LSD should be purchased from a reputable source and tested for purity.

4. **Have a trusted, sober sitter who is trusted and experienced in supporting psychedelic sessions.** A sitter's job is to be present with the person taking a given substance to help ensure a safe and positive experience. Having a trusted, sober guide will reduce the chances of a bad trip. This person should be someone that the LSD-taker feels comfortable with and trusts. They should have a deep knowledge of psychedelics and the safety guidelines for use.

When it comes to LSD experiences, set and setting are everything. Set refers to the psychological state of mind of the person taking the drug, while setting refers to the physical and social environment in which the trip is taking place. Both factors can heavily influence the nature of an LSD experience. For example, if someone is feeling anxious or depressed before taking LSD, they are more likely to have a bad trip. Likewise, if the environment is loud and chaotic, this can also lead to a negative experience. On the other hand, if the person is in a good mood and the setting is peaceful and supportive, then the trip is more likely to be positive. By taking the set and setting into consideration, it is possible to reduce the chances of having a bad trip on LSD.

BEFORE DECIDING TO USE LSD, THE FOLLOWING FACTORS SHOULD BE CONSIDERED:

1. **Mindset**: What is the person's mood like at the time of the trip? Have they prepared and thoroughly researched benefits and risks? What does the person expect to gain from the experience? A long-range mindset should also be

considered. If the person has previous traumas in their life, they may resurface during the trip.
2. **Physical Setting**: Is the person surrounded by people they trust, including an experienced guide or sitter? Is the person indoors in a therapeutic or clinical environment? Are they outdoors in a natural setting? Experiencing a trip in a clinical setting or alongside an experienced guide will produce a much different experience than tripping at a party or club.
3. **Comfort**: Some people prefer to experience a trip in darkness and with evocative music. Others prefer to experience a trip outdoors while connecting with nature. Much of the comfort factors will depend on the person's individual preferences.

HOW MUCH LSD IS SAFE TO CONSUME?

The appropriate amount of LSD to take is dependent on the desired outcome. Dosage can vary depending on the type of LSD as well as where it is sourced from but generally falls into one of two categories: a full dose or a microdose.

There is no set dose of LSD that will guarantee a psychedelic experience. The amount required will differ depending on clinical versus recreational use, with a full dose ranging from 25µg to 200µg Holze et al. (2021). The effects of a full dose are felt between 100µg-200µg. When taking LSD for the first time, it is recommended to start with a lower dose in order to see how much is needed to produce the desired effects. Everyone's brain chemistry is different, so what may be a full dose for one person may not have the same effect on another person. Experimentation is key in finding the right dosage. Too little LSD may not produce the desired effect, while too much could lead to an unpleasant experience. Therefore, it is important to start low and increase the dosage gradually until the desired effects are achieved.

Microdosing is an alternative option for those who are not looking to experience a trip but would like to experience the health-related benefits of LSD. Microdosing has allowed people to explore some of the benefits of LSD without the fear and stigma that is typically associated with it. When done correctly, microdosing allows people to have a safe, therapeutic experience with perceived lasting benefits. Typically, a microdose is somewhere between one-tenth and one-twentieth of a full dose.

WHAT DOES AN LSD TRIP FEEL LIKE?

A person's unique body chemistry, as well as set and setting, plays a major role in how they experience the effects of LSD. Some people may have a stronger resistance to the drug and will experience less intense visions than others. As previously stated, many factors contribute to a personal experience with LSD, including dose, mindset, setting, and personal body chemistry. Some people may have a higher resistance to the drug and won't experience visual effects as intensely as others.

Some people report that LSD helped them gain insight into themselves, their lives, and the nature of the universe. Steve Jobs, the founder of Apple, has been quoted as saying that his experience with LSD was "one of the most profound experiences" of his life. Some people associate psychedelic substances with greater spiritual awareness. When the moods of both the person taking LSD and those around them are buoyant or contented, the LSD experience can be highly enjoyable.

One of the most difficult things about a trip is that it's impossible to know when a challenging trip might occur (although taking the safety precautions mentioned above can greatly reduce the chances of challenging experiences).

HOW LONG DO THE EFFECTS OF LSD TAKE TO KICK IN, AND HOW LONG WILL A TRIP LAST?

The effects of LSD vary from person to person, with some people feeling effects as soon as 10 minutes after ingestion and others taking up to 2 hours to feel anything (Jarvik, Abramson, and Hirsch, 1955). Pharmacological measures such as "peak plasma level," or the time at which the most LSD is in your bloodstream is in the range of 90 minutes after ingestion, and the "half-life," or time at which the blood level is one half of the dose taken, is about 2.5 hours (Dolder et al., 2017). This means that the effects of LSD can last for several hours after ingestion.

Interestingly, the subjective effects will "peak" around 3-4 hours after ingestion, and effects can last anywhere from 8-16 hours. To add to LSD's long duration, even when it wears off, it is sometimes hard to fall asleep. For this reason, one should plan to take LSD on a day when there are no other responsibilities and there is no need to drive anywhere.

On a trip, the person's perception of time can extend and distort, making them feel like they're on a forever-long journey. People who know this ahead of time—and can remember that they WILL eventually return to their normal state of consciousness—are less likely to experience anxiety or a bad trip.

A POWERFUL SUBSTANCE TO BE USED WITH CARE & RESPECT

LSD is a powerful psychedelic substance that can induce profound changes in perception, sensation, and cognition. When used in a responsible and safe manner, it has the potential to help people have deep personal insights, spiritual experiences, and enhanced creativity. However, LSD is also a very potent drug, and it should be respected as such. It should never be taken carelessly or without proper preparation. Always obtain psychedelics from a trusted source and test for purity. And it is always best to have access to a trusted and experienced professional when using LSD or any other psychedelic substance. With proper respect and precautions, LSD can be a powerful tool for personal growth and transformation.

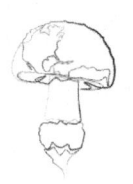

REFERENCES:

- Dyck, E. (2006). 'Hitting Highs at Rock Bottom': LSD Treatment for Alcoholism, 1950–1970. *Social History of Medicine, 19*(2), 313-329. doi:10.1093/shm/hkl039
- Krebs, T. S., & Johansen, P. (2012). Lysergic acid diethylamide (LSD) for alcoholism: meta-analysis of randomized controlled trials. *Journal of psychopharmacology (Oxford, England), 26*(7), 994-1002. doi:10.1177/0269881112439253
- Liechti, M. E. (2017). Modern Clinical Research on LSD. *Neuropsychopharmacology : official publication of the American College of Neuropsychopharmacology, 42*(11), 2114-2127. doi:10.1038/npp.2017.86
- Nichols, D. E. (2016). Psychedelics. *Pharmacol Rev, 68*(2), 264-355. doi:10.1124/pr.115.011478

- Schechter, M. D. (1998). 'Candyflipping': synergistic discriminative effect of LSD and MDMA. *Eur J Pharmacol, 341*(2-3), 131-134. doi:10.1016/s0014-2999(97)01473-8
- Schmid, Y., Gasser, P., Oehen, P., & Liechti, M. (2020). Acute subjective effects in LSD- and MDMA-assisted psychotherapy. *Journal of Psychopharmacology, 35*, 026988112095960. doi:10.1177/0269881120959604
- Schmid, Y., & Liechti, M. E. (2018). Long-lasting subjective effects of LSD in normal subjects. *Psychopharmacology, 235*(2), 535-545. doi:10.1007/s00213-017-4733-3
- Smigielski, L., Scheidegger, M., Kometer, M., & Vollenweider, F. X. (2019). Psilocybin-assisted mindfulness training modulates self-consciousness and brain default mode network connectivity with lasting effects. *Neuroimage, 196*, 207-215. doi:10.1016/j.neuroimage.2019.04.009

TWENTY-SEVEN
GUIDE TO MICRODOSING LSD
AMELIA WALSH

MEDICALLY REVIEWED BY DR. LYNN-MARIE MORSKI, MD, JD

Psychedelics have been used for centuries in various cultures for healing and spiritual purposes. In recent years, there has been a renewed interest in their potential medicinal benefits. Microdosing is a practice whereby people take small doses of psychedelics on a regular basis in order to achieve specific therapeutic goals.

The appeal of microdosing lies in its potential to produce subtle yet profound changes in mood, cognition, and creativity. Lysergic acid diethylamide (LSD) has demonstrated positive effects for psychotherapeutic purposes at full dosage, but many people wonder if smaller, more consistent applications might offer different benefits (Fuentes, Fonseca, Elices, Farré, & Torrens, 2020). Additionally, microdosing has been associated with enhanced cognitive function and improved creativity and productivity. Given the promising preliminary evidence, it is likely that more research will be conducted on the potential benefits of microdosing in the future.

WHAT IS MICRODOSING?

The term microdosing refers to taking a very small, sub-perceptual amount of a psychedelic substance on a planned schedule to benefit from certain effects while avoiding impaired functionality. Advocates of microdosing believe that by taking a very small amount of a substance on a regular basis, they can reap the benefits of the substance without experiencing the impairments that come with taking a larger dose. While there is not yet sufficient scientific evidence to support this claim, many people who have tried microdosing report feeling more energetic, creative, and productive.

Others claim that microdosing improves their mood, alleviates anxiety, helps with cognitive function, bolsters creativity, and elevates the capacity to empathize with others. Others have reported reduced dependency on caffeine or declined inclination to consume alcohol and other illicit drugs like cocaine.

However, research to investigate these claims has been insufficient and somewhat inconclusive. Most of the touted personal benefits of microdosing are self-reported or anecdotal, leaving many questions about other factors that could influence individual results from microdosing.

There is a possibility that some people who experience benefits from microdosing experience a placebo effect. In a placebo-controlled study on microdosing with almost 200 participants conducted by Imperial College, both the placebo group and those who microdosed psychedelics reported a similar rate of positive psychological effects (Szigeti et al., 2021). Contrastingly, a 2018 study of 38 participants by Leiden University found that convergent (coming up with a well-defined solution to a problem) and divergent thinking (creative thinking) performance improved while fluid intelligence remained unaffected (Prochazkova et al., 2018). A 2020 double-blind controlled study from Maastricht University with 24 participants found that microdosing reduced their pain perception (Kuypers, 2020).

HOW DO YOU MICRODOSE LSD?

Microdosing remains a largely understudied phenomenon, and as a result, there is no official recommended dosage or frequency. However, there are some general guidelines that have been shared by the psychedelic community and substance experts. These guidelines suggest that the ideal dosage for different individuals may vary depending on the substance being used, the individual's weight and tolerance, and the goals they are hoping to achieve.

James Fadiman, a clinical psychologist and author with expertise in the exploratory use of psychedelic substances, has been one of the leading sources of information about how to experiment with microdosing. He recommends a microdose that is one-tenth of a typical dose; this equates to about 10-20 micrograms of LSD (Fadiman, 2011; Fadiman & Korb, 2019).

It's recommended to be conservative in the beginning, as taking too much may result in unintentional, inconvenient, or unsafe impairment. A general rule with ingesting any dose or type of psychedelic is to "start low, go slow" to determine how the body will react to the particular medicine. The best way to avoid taking too much is to properly measure each dose and maintain a record of when and how much LSD has been consumed.

Common practice is to have a "dose day" every three days, taking two days to rest between them. Many who microdose LSD report adhering to this schedule for a period of two weeks several times a year as a form of occasional maintenance.

SIDE EFFECTS AND RISKS OF MICRODOSING LSD

The effects of LSD can range from immensely meaningful and positive to challenging, frightening, or even disturbing. Though the small dose is not likely to cause overwhelming, negative hallucinations, there is a lack of research to determine the possibility of negative psychological reactions to LSD when microdosing.

It is not recommended for people with a personal or family history of psychosis to use psychedelics like LSD. While rare, there have been reports of "flashbacks," where a person continues to recall certain unpleasant hallucinations that occurred while taking LSD. Because of the sub-perceptual dosage used to microdose psychedelics, this phenomenon is highly unlikely but still ought to be a consideration (particularly for those at risk of mania and psychotic episodes).

Some physical side effects of LSD may include dilated pupils and elevated blood pressure, and/or heart rate. People with heart conditions are advised not to use LSD as it can cause additional health complications that may become dangerous. Even in small doses, LSD has the potential to cause anxiety or physical discomfort.

MICRODOSING LSD: IS IT FOR YOU?

Many people who advocate for microdosing claim that it can help with a variety of issues, such as depression, anxiety, and chronic pain. Although there is not yet sufficient scientific evidence to support these claims, some preliminary studies have shown promise. However, it is important to note that most of the evidence for the benefits of microdosing is anecdotal or based on personal experiences. As a result, it is difficult to say definitively whether microdosing is effective. Additionally, because LSD is a Schedule I drug in the United States, it is illegal to use for personal reasons. If you are considering microdosing, it is important to do plenty of research first and be aware of the risks involved.

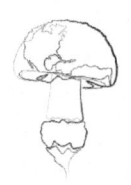

REFERENCES:

- Fadiman, J. (2011). *The psychedelic explorer's guide: Safe, therapeutic, and sacred journeys*: Simon and Schuster.
- Fadiman, J., & Korb, S. (2019). Might Microdosing Psychedelics Be Safe and Beneficial? An Initial Exploration. *Journal of Psychoactive Drugs, 51*(2), 118-122. doi:10.1080/02791072.2019.1593561
- Kuypers, K. P. C. (2020). The therapeutic potential of microdosing psychedelics in depression. *Ther Adv Psychopharmacol, 10*, 2045125320950567. doi:10.1177/2045125320950567
- Prochazkova, L., Lippelt, D. P., Colzato, L. S., Kuchar, M., Sjoerds, Z., & Hommel, B. (2018). Exploring the effect of microdosing psychedelics on creativity in an open-label natural setting. *Psychopharmacology, 235*(12), 3401-3413. doi:10.1007/s00213-018-5049-7
- Szigeti, B., Kartner, L., Blemings, A., Rosas, F., Feilding, A., Nutt, D. J., . . . Erritzoe, D. (2021). Self-blinding citizen science to explore psychedelic microdosing. *Elife, 10*. doi:10.7554/eLife.62878

PART EIGHT
SAN PEDRO AND PEYOTE

"In consciousness dwells the wondrous, with it man attains the realm beyond the material, and the Peyote tells us, where to find it."

Antonin Artaud

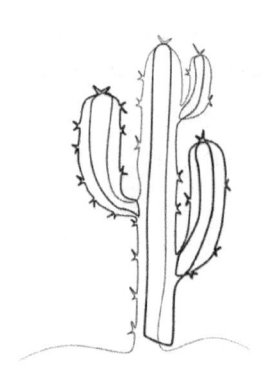

TWENTY-EIGHT
A BEGINNER'S GUIDE TO SAN PEDRO
KATIE STONE, MA

MEDICALLY REVIEWED BY DR. DAVID COX, PHD, ABPP

San Pedro cactus, also known as *huachuma* (wa-choo'-ma), is one of several cacti that produce the alkaloid mescaline, the psychoactive compound that inspired the term *psychedelic* in the first place (Tanne, 2004).

San Pedro cactus is a columnar cactus that grows in the Andes mountains. It is prized as an ornamental and landscape plant due in part to its massive and short-lived blooms. The cactus' flowers only open at night and just for a few days — sometimes unfurling for only a single night before beginning to decay. Their fragrance attracts nighttime pollinators like bats, and the cactus produces fruits after fertilization.

Under the invasion of the Spanish armies and missionaries in the 17th century, who condemned it as a form of devil worship, the huachuma cactus became known colloquially as *San Pedro* or St. Peter. The medicine has been used in ceremonies for millennia by Andean cultures, alongside coca, datura, and tobacco, to support physical health and spiritual well-being (Carod-Artal & Vázquez-Cabrera, 2006). Incredibly, the ceremony still remains an important part of Peruvian culture. In recent decades, Westerners have begun traveling to Peru to participate in authentic and legal San Pedro ceremonies.

LEGAL STATUS OF SAN PEDRO

In the United States, the San Pedro cactus itself is legal. Commercial nurseries and hobbyist gardeners sell San Pedro regularly. As with all naturally occurring psychedelics, mescaline is *biosynthesized* and naturally produced by a living organism. It is illegal to isolate mescaline from San Pedro or to prepare it for consumption.

Before the passage of the Controlled Substances Act in 1970, mescaline was used alongside psychotherapy and demonstrated therapeutic potential (Uthaug et al., 2021). After it was classified as a Schedule 1 drug, it became illegal to use, process, cultivate, or sell mescaline extracted from San Pedro and other mescaline-containing cacti.

Mescaline is regulated as an illicit substance around the world, and transporting cacti might be illegal. However, there are varying exemptions for research, religious purposes, and hobbyist horticulture in several countries around the world. San Pedro's use in healing ceremonies is legal for travelers visiting Peru.

As drug policies continue to evolve, it is conceivable that mescaline could re-emerge as a therapeutic tool. It is currently being used in one psychedelic clinical trial investigating the comparative effects of classical psychedelics and was used recently in a comprehensive hallucinogenic study looking at the effects of psychedelics on mood.

PHARMACOLOGY OF SAN PEDRO

Beyond mescaline itself, San Pedro contains dozens of alkaloids that interact with the body on a multitude of levels. The cactus has been used in folk healing for over 8,000 years, both for physical healing for indigestion, burns, and oedema and for supernatural diseases including *susto, vaho de agua, mal aire, mal hecho, shuka*, conditions, which traditional healers attribute to spiritual causes (Shetty, Rana, & Preetham, 2012). Today, its extracts are used for stimulating the nervous system as well as regulating blood pressure, hunger, sleep, and thirst (Franco-Molina et al., 2003). It also is being studied for the treatment of non-insulin-dependent diabetes mellitus (Frati et al., 1990).

The primary psychoactive compound is mescaline, considered a classical psychedelic because it binds to the 5HT2A serotonin receptor. It also shows an affinity for the 5-HT2C receptor in the brain and causes physiological impacts that can leave a person in an altered state for hours. It increases activity in the right side of the brain's striatum limbic system. Cross-tolerance has been shown to occur within this classification of drugs and is restored after 3-4 days of abstinence (Dinis-Oliveira, Pereira, & da Silva, 2019).

Mescaline is *biosynthesized*, meaning it is created naturally by biologically living organisms. The distribution of mescaline within San Pedro varies, and so do its physiological impacts. Mescaline has a low potency, and the volume required for research studies can be significant (Kovacic & Somanathan, 2009). It's available as a research chemical and is usually in the form of a whitish powder.

The body reacts to mescaline with an increase in stress hormones, causing pupil dilation, perspiration, hypertension, nausea, and increased temperature. Muscle strength temporarily weakens, reflexes and coordination are diminished, and people experience intestinal and sometimes uterine contractions (Kovacic & Somanathan, 2009).

Mescaline is the longest-studied psychedelic compound in terms of its chemistry, and several synthetic mescaline alternatives exist—but clinical trials are uncommon when compared to other psychedelics with greater potency (Jay, 2019). Early research at the beginning of the 20th century featured mescaline-induced mind states to study psychosis and theories of schizophrenia (Guttmann & Maclay, 1936).

More recently, the US-based chemist Alexander Shulgin used mescaline as a starting point for synthesizing dozens of experimental psychedelic compounds. In fact, Shulgin published a psychedelic cult classic focusing on these compounds, called *PiHKAL: A Love Story*, an acronym for "phenethylamines I have known and loved" (Shulgin, Shulgin, & Nichols, 1991). Mescaline has also emerged as a potential candidate for microdosing, although questions remain regarding whether microdosing psychedelics work any better than microdosing a placebo (Polito & Stevenson, 2019; Szigeti et al., 2021).

Mescaline is a molecular alkaloid and is considered a classic psychedelic, like psilocybin and LSD, but it is in a different classification of drugs called phenethylamines. It can be smoked or insufflated (snorted) but is typically consumed orally. In the case of San Pedro, it is usually consumed as a decoction prepared from boiling water and sliced cactus.

Mescaline is quickly absorbed by the digestive system, and it reaches various organs throughout your body, specifically the liver and kidneys. It is not yet fully understood how the drug is metabolized, but some believe that different parts of the body may process mescaline through different localized routes.

SAN PEDRO DOSING

San Pedro is typically ingested as a dried powder or tea made from the cacti. Dosing is imprecise if using a live cactus, as the distribution of mescaline is not consistent throughout all parts of the cactus. An average dose of pure mescaline is 20-500 mg. The onset will begin within 1-3 hours depending on the metabolization rate, and may last up to 10-12 hours.

Typically, an active dose of mescaline will last under 24 hours, with visual effects averaging around 10-12 hours. People experience distortions in sensory stimuli, like sounds and colors, and even experience synesthesia. While intoxication can occur, it is reportedly unlikely for a fatality to result from San Pedro consumption alone (Dinis-Oliveira et al., 2019). While there have been mescaline deaths reported in animal studies, these occurred at a level of mescaline toxicity that is unlikely to happen in a San Pedro ceremony (Kovacic & Somanathan, 2009).

San Pedro contains more alkaloids than just mescaline. It is thought that these alkaloids work together in an entourage effect; however, little research has been conducted. San Pedro also has various concentrations of other compounds, including anhalonidine, hordenine, and tyramine. Consuming mescaline-containing cacti, rather than pure mescaline, will result in a different experience, mainly because the dosing will be imprecise and may last longer than with other cacti.

While there are no significant studies to verify mescaline distribution throughout San Pedro, it is generally thought that the external green tissue contains more mescaline than the internal white tissue near the center.

ARE THERE RISKS ASSOCIATED WITH USING SAN PEDRO?

It is important to note that all psychedelics are potentially risky for people with pre-existing medical conditions, especially those dealing with hypertension or heart disease, and mental health risks may be more significant in those who have had a history of psychosis. Mescaline itself has low risk — though there are rare exceptions. Mescaline is considered the least potent classical psychedelic

(Kovacic & Somanathan, 2009). San Pedro is thought by some to be among the safest psychoactive plants — but traditional ceremonies might involve additional plants with toxicity potential (like datura), and mescaline-based synthetics can be harmful.

Synthesized mescaline is not a prolific substance among people who use psychedelics, but people who microdose mescaline might use synthetics. There are potentially lethal novel psychedelic substances derived from mescaline called NBOMes (*N*-Benzylphenethylamine). These synthetics share the same unique classification of drugs called phenethylamines and may produce similar effects but carry a much higher risk of fatality (Andreasen et al., 2015).

People who seek mescaline from illicit sources may inadvertently encounter a potentially toxic synthetic instead. Any person or provider working with mescaline should make sure to test the substance to confirm it is not dangerous. While testing kits are usually legal, mescaline is not. People who microdose isolated mescaline should be cautious of contaminants.

San Pedro is not recommended for pregnant people because mescaline has been shown to cause uterine contractions, however, some mescaline-containing substances have been used by indigenous groups to maintain reproductive health.

Mescaline is rapidly metabolized in the liver, and for this reason, there could be a potential for complications for those with liver conditions. Early studies involving mescaline and ethanol withdrawal did not demonstrate complications or life-threatening symptoms — but the real risks are unknown without clinical trials (Dinis-Oliveira et al., 2019).

Though mescaline is used as a research chemical, it is not typically studied in clinical trials for toxicity, nor is San Pedro. Anecdotally, the additional plants used in San Pedro ceremonies, such as the potentially lethal *datura*, are more likely to cause complications than the mescaline-containing cacti themselves.

Currently, there are no clinical studies investigating the safety of San Pedro. But it is considered relatively safe — so long as one does not have any pre-existing health conditions of the heart or primary organs.

Working with well-referenced and experienced healers during ceremonies is essential for minimizing risk in a San Pedro ceremony. So too is communicating any pre-existing health concerns with the provider, especially those requiring medication.

Because mescaline can interfere with some antidepressants containing MAOIs, a provider might advise tapering off these medications. However, this can be risky on its own and should only be done under medical supervision.

HOW TO PREPARE FOR A SAN PEDRO EXPERIENCE

Preparing for a San Pedro experience will vary depending on whether it takes place in a traditional ceremony or not. If you are participating in a traditional ceremony, your guide will likely ask you to abstain from alcohol, meat, and rich foods in the days leading up to the event. You may also be asked to meditate or perform other spiritually-oriented practices. It is important to follow these instructions carefully, as they will help to ensure that your experience is safe and beneficial. In a traditional ceremony, the local healer, sometimes called a *Yachakkuna*, will consume San Pedro as well.

An altar called a *mesa* would likely be created before the San Pedro ceremony, featuring meaningful items collected by the Yachakkuna over time. Flowers, stones, and other objects are precisely placed to help shape the energetic container of the experience and transfer power to the healer. Depending on the Yachakkuna and the ceremony's intention, they may offer a traditional sacrifice (guinea pig) in exchange for divining healing insight.

As with any psychedelic experience, preparation includes intention setting and self-reflection. In the case of San Pedro, it is also advised to arrive in a spirit of gratitude and reverence for the plant teacher that makes healing possible.

EXPERIENCING A SAN PEDRO TRIP: WHAT TO EXPECT

Using isolated, synthetic mescaline will likely result in a slightly different trip than if using San Pedro. As a living organism, every cactus grows a little differently and will present varying concentrations of alkaloids, including mescaline, ranging from 150 mg to 1.2g of mescaline per 50g of dried cactus. Whereas mescaline might be administered according to body weight, San Pedro cannot be dosed as precisely.

The San Pedro cactus might be presented as a powder ground from dried cactus or sliced into wedges and boiled in water as a decoction. In traditional ceremonies, the participants receive a smaller dose than the healer and may not even experience psychoactive effects. Depending on what the Yachakkuna determines is the cause of disease, additional plants may be prepared for treatment.

The tea reportedly tastes bitter and unpleasant, and many people tend to feel nauseous and vomit after drinking. The effects usually begin between 15-40 minutes after consuming the tea, with the experience building in intensity over the first 1-3 hours before reaching the peak around hour three or four.

San Pedro effects can be felt for 12-14 hours, depending on the dose ingested and the person's physiology. The most active part of the experience can last for two hours, with people reporting a relatively easy comedown and an overall experience more similar to

MDMA than LSD. During the post-peak period, it can be a good idea to reflect on what you've experienced and start to think about post-trip integration. This is when many people find it helpful to journal or talk to someone about their trip. Integration can be a key part of making sure that you find value and meaning in your experience.

HISTORY OF SAN PEDRO

While the emergence of mescaline use in the West is one of the psychedelic culture's most defining moments, another, more ancient story places the mescaline-containing cactus San Pedro, or *huachuma*, among the oldest recorded visionary plants used in human history.

The Chavin culture is named in reference to an ancient religious site called Chavin de Huantar. The place was a center of life, commerce, and technology for an ancient Andean society that spanned a large geographic region. Residual *Echinopsis pachanoi* cactus elements have been observed in several ancient sites, with the earliest fossil evidence of San Pedro use dating back 8,000 years.

Chavin culture developed specific artistic aesthetics evident in ceramics, sculpture, and architecture — and much of these aesthetics and symbology are thought to be inspired by the use of San Pedro, or *huachuma.* In the Quechua language, the term translates to *removing the head*.

Interestingly, San Pedro grows in the highlands, but the Chavin de Huantar's site is located beyond this cacti's typical range. It has been suggested that this ancient culture began to cultivate the mescaline-containing cactus, effectively domesticating it for sacred use.

Evident in sculpture and artwork throughout the site, *huachuma* was transported there for ritual and group ceremonies. Carvings at

Chavin de Huantar reveal God-like figures, and images of people consuming San Pedro and transforming into jaguars and other animals. Archeological evidence reveals ceramic containers with pouring lips shaped like the cactus, suggesting to some archeologists that these vessels were ritually significant and meant to serve and share traditional San Pedro tea.

As Christianity and the Spanish conquistadors began pushing into the Andean homelands, the indigenous healing rituals and religious ceremonies tied to *huachuma* were hidden and blended syncretically with settler religious ideologies. The cactus and traditional rituals survived the onslaught of colonization but emerged as San Pedro, or St. Peter, who guards the gates to heaven — a nod to *huachuma,* which also opens the gates to the spiritual realm.

In a traditional ceremony, healers called *Yachakkuna* are responsible for carrying on the lineage and caring for the community's health. The Yachakkuna consumes the mescaline-containing cactus to help gain insight into a participant's illness. In this way, San Pedro works as a diagnostic tool for identifying the causes of disease, whether physical or spiritual.

San Pedro is used for more than diagnosis, but also for spiritual well-being. Traditional healers use the San Pedro rituals to facilitate clearing emotional energies. Participants frequently experience spiritual healing in the form of tears.

San Pedro has long been regarded as a beneficial protector of marriage and family relationships and is often planted near homes. Unlike other mescaline-containing cacti, San Pedro is not a legally protected religious sacrament.

ETHICAL CONCERNS WHEN USING SAN PEDRO

There are a few ethical implications related to the consumption of San Pedro worth mentioning.

First, this species is frequently recommended as the more ethical option among mescaline cacti — because peyote is a threatened species with considerable cultural baggage surrounding its use. As it stands today in the US, the Native American Church has an exemption to use peyote as a religious sacrament; however, the use of peyote by those who are not members of federally recognized tribes is illegal.

A San Pedro ceremony may be unethical if the facilitator illegitimately claims to be from a specified lineage, especially when charging money and profiting off an indigenous culture's traditional knowledge. This is different from sitting in a ceremony with friends and family.

It is common for San Pedro to be used outside of traditional ceremonies without crossing ethical boundaries — ethical use means this is done with a healthy respect to the plant teacher, the participants, and the ritual space.

Another ethical consideration surrounding San Pedro involves researchers and practitioners. As drug policies continue to evolve, San Pedro will likely be studied in greater detail, both from a pharmacological standpoint and within psychotherapy, as a component of psychedelic-assisted therapy.

To ensure that San Pedro's use remains ethical, it is essential to start considering the implications of applying the Nagoya Protocol to any current and future research involving this healing cactus. The psychoactive compound in San Pedro is only one of the dozens of active chemicals produced by the cactus, and the entourage effect of these alkaloids with mescaline has not been studied yet.

Established by the United Nations in 2010, the full name of the agreement reads "The *Nagoya Protocol on Access to Genetic Resources and the Fair and Equitable Sharing of Benefits Arising from their Utilization.*" Said simply, the Nagoya Protocol aims to protect traditional ecological knowledge (TEK) from exploitation, which has historically been common.

In the case of San Pedro, exploitation might look like attempts to patent traditional healing modalities, such as communal ceremony or the antimicrobial peptides found in the cactus. Because San Pedro also has additional medicinal properties, the cactus is also at risk of biopiracy from medical researchers. An ethical future for San Pedro will need to keep indigenous sovereignty in mind.

HOW TO CHOOSE A SAN PEDRO PROVIDER

When working with any psychedelic, it's important to have experienced and qualified facilitators. It's important to note that in traditional ceremonies the healer might ingest San Pedro as well, though this is not recommended for providers working outside of the ritual environment. Instead, a sober sitter or guide who is well experienced with San Pedro dosing is ideal.

Ideally, a center and provider will require the completion of a medical intake form to identify any pre-existing health conditions. The provider might also incorporate other plants in a ceremony and should provide information on all plants used. While San Pedro is generally safe, there should be a protocol to handle any emergencies that might arise. If a center or provider is not asking questions or taking precautionary measures to ensure safety, it might be better to look elsewhere.

San Pedro ceremonies are legal in Peru. A psychedelic tourism industry has emerged, featuring retreat centers that offer massage, workshops, group therapy, and potentially additional plant medicines such as ayahuasca. Depending on one's desires, a multi-day or multi-week retreat might be ideal. Be sure to allow room for post-trip rest and integration before returning to your day-to-day life.

Sometimes San Pedro retreat centers and practitioners might prioritize profit over care. Before committing to a retreat center, people should conduct personal research to get a sense of how previous participants felt about their experiences and their specific providers.

Searching through social media pages, online forums, and general searches about any history of scams or adverse health events will help ensure a safe experience. And while a friend's recommendation is valid, it should always be backed up with research before making a final decision when choosing a San Pedro retreat center.

A final consideration is cost. Meals might be included in the price or might have an additional charge. Some centers are more remote and inaccessible than others, and travel from the airport may or may not be covered. Medical travel insurance is recommended if a complication does arise, but it does not typically cover transportation to emergency medical centers.

SAN PEDRO'S HEALING POTENTIAL: HOW DOES MESCALINE SUPPORT WELLBEING?

While mescaline has been studied longer than any other psychedelic, the therapeutic potentials of San Pedro have yet to be studied in clinical trials.

Like other classic psychedelics, mescaline-containing cacti can induce mystical experiences capable of catalyzing profound and lasting personality changes (Carhart-Harris & Goodwin, 2017). Common mental health ailments like depression, PTSD, addictive behaviors, and anxiety disorders are all potentially treatable with these psychedelics.

From an indigenous perspective of illness, all disease has a spiritual component that can be treated to heal the physical element. Mescaline-containing cacti like San Pedro have been used in healing ceremonies for millennia, not only for spiritual ailments but also for physical diseases like cancer and paralysis and as topical treatments for inflammation and pain. But even in these cases, the spiritual aspect of the San Pedro ceremony plays a part in the healing process.

Cultural beliefs and group settings may also play a role in healing with San Pedro. Psychedelics taken in traditional settings and in nature have demonstrated enhanced therapeutic potential, especially with long-term integration. With this in mind, it is possible that aspects of the traditional San Pedro ceremony, held in a naturalistic setting, can uniquely complement psychotherapy by maximizing the psychological benefits of nature-relatedness — but until thorough research is conducted, these claims cannot be verified.

Drawing from the long history of psychedelic medicine ceremonies, some researchers today suggest it is worth revisiting this enduring power of communal ritual used in combination with mind-altering psychedelics (Anderson et al., 2020; Trope et al., 2019). In this regard, San Pedro might one day be an easy-to-grow, safe-to-use option for community-based group therapy processes.

SAN PEDRO HAS THE POTENTIAL TO GROW BEYOND RELIGIOUS AND TRADITIONAL SETTINGS

San Pedro, a naturally occurring plant that grows quickly and abundantly in its natural habitat, currently has no risk of extinction like other sacred plants. Its use goes back thousands of years, but unlike peyote, it isn't currently a legal part of any religion or closed spiritual tradition.

Traditional ceremonies are lawfully held in Peru, and some people use San Pedro in non-traditional settings. While there is not a great deal of research on San Pedro specifically, there is clinical evidence of the benefits of its primary psychoactive compound, mescaline, which is considered the first-ever substance to be called *psychedelic*.

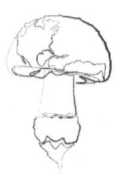

REFERENCES:

- Anderson, B. T., Danforth, A., Daroff, R., Stauffer, C., Ekman, E., Agin-Liebes, G., . . . Mitchell, J. (2020). Psilocybin-assisted group therapy for demoralized older long-term AIDS survivor men: An open-label safety and feasibility pilot study. *EClinicalMedicine, 27*, 100538.
- Andreasen, M. F., Telving, R., Rosendal, I., Eg, M. B., Hasselstrøm, J. B., & Andersen, L. V. (2015). A fatal poisoning involving 25C-NBOMe. *Forensic Science International, 251*, e1-e8. doi:https://doi.org/10.1016/j.forsciint.2015.03.012
- Carhart-Harris, R. L., & Goodwin, G. M. (2017). The Therapeutic Potential of Psychedelic Drugs: Past, Present, and Future. *Neuropsychopharmacology, 42*(11), 2105-2113. doi:10.1038/npp.2017.84
- Carod-Artal, F. J., & Vázquez-Cabrera, C. B. (2006). [Mescaline and the San Pedro cactus ritual: archaeological and ethnographic evidence in northern Peru]. *Rev Neurol, 42*(8), 489-498.
- Dinis-Oliveira, R. J., Pereira, C. L., & da Silva, D. D. (2019). Pharmacokinetic and Pharmacodynamic Aspects of Peyote and Mescaline: Clinical and Forensic Repercussions. *Curr*

- *Mol Pharmacol, 12*(3), 184-194. doi:10.2174/1874467211666181010154139
- Franco-Molina, M., Gomez-Flores, R., Tamez-Guerra, P., Tamez-Guerra, R., Castillo-Leon, L., & Rodríguez-Padilla, C. (2003). In vitro immunopotentiating properties and tumour cell toxicity induced by Lophophora williamsii (peyote) cactus methanolic extract. *Phytother Res, 17*(9), 1076-1081. doi:10.1002/ptr.1313
- Frati, A. C., Cordillo, B. E., Altamirano, P., Ariza, C. R., Cortés-Franco, R., & Chavez-Negrete, A. (1990). Acute hypoglycemic effect of Opuntia streptacantha Lemaire in NIDDM. *Diabetes Care, 13*(4), 455-456.
- Guttmann, E., & Maclay, W. S. (1936). Mescalin and Depersonalization: Therapeutic Experiments. *The Journal of neurology and psychopathology, 16*(63), 193-212. doi:10.1136/jnnp.s1-16.63.193
- Jay, M. (2019). Mescaline : a global history of the first psychedelic. Retrieved from https://www.degruyter.com/isbn/9780300245080
- Kovacic, P., & Somanathan, R. (2009). Novel, unifying mechanism for mescaline in the central nervous system: electrochemistry, catechol redox metabolite, receptor, cell signaling and structure activity relationships. *Oxidative medicine and cellular longevity, 2*(4), 181-190. doi:10.4161/oxim.2.4.9380
- Polito, V., & Stevenson, R. J. (2019). A systematic study of microdosing psychedelics. *PloS one, 14*(2), e0211023-e0211023. doi:10.1371/journal.pone.0211023
- Shetty, A. A., Rana, M. K., & Preetham, S. P. (2012). Cactus: a medicinal food. *Journal of food science and technology, 49*(5), 530-536. doi:10.1007/s13197-011-0462-5
- Shulgin, A., Shulgin, A., & Nichols, D. (1991). Phenethylamines I have known and loved: a chemical love

story. *Transform Pr. USA*.
- Szigeti, B., Kartner, L., Blemings, A., Rosas, F., Feilding, A., Nutt, D. J., . . . Erritzoe, D. (2021). Self-blinding citizen science to explore psychedelic microdosing. *Elife, 10*. doi:10.7554/eLife.62878
- Tanne, J. H. (2004). Humphry Osmond. *BMJ : British Medical Journal, 328*(7441), 713-713. Retrieved from https://www.ncbi.nlm.nih.gov/pmc/articles/PMC381240/
- Trope, A., Anderson, B. T., Hooker, A. R., Glick, G., Stauffer, C., & Woolley, J. D. (2019). Psychedelic-Assisted Group Therapy: A Systematic Review. *Journal of Psychoactive Drugs, 51*(2), 174-188. doi:10.1080/02791072.2019.1593559
- Uthaug, M. V., Davis, A. K., Haas, T. F., Davis, D., Dolan, S. B., Lancelotta, R., . . . Ramaekers, J. G. (2021). The epidemiology of mescaline use: Pattern of use, motivations for consumption, and perceived consequences, benefits, and acute and enduring subjective effects. *Journal of Psychopharmacology, 36*(3), 309-320. doi:10.1177/02698811211013583

TWENTY-NINE
WHY PEYOTE SUSTAINABILITY MATTERS
ALICE DE WITT

When most people think of sustainability, they tend to think of environmental issues. However, sustainability is also about sustaining cultures and traditions. For the Native American Church (NAC), sustainability of peyote means a discussion about both environmental concerns *and* sustaining the use of peyote as a religious sacrament. Peyote is a key part of the NAC's ceremonies, and it is also a source of mescaline, a *psychedelic* compound that has been used for therapeutic purposes. As such, there is a natural alliance between supporting psychedelic therapy and supporting peyote conservation efforts. By working collectively, we can help to ensure that both the environment and traditional cultures are able to thrive.

Without immediate action and intention, there are serious risks of peyote disappearing in the United States. In Texas, the sacrament is considered to be endangered at the local level. Peyote sustainability is possible, but only if people consider the ethical issues surrounding peyote and make it a priority to support the cultures that steward this medicine.

While some traditional psychedelic ceremonies are open to all and invite participants, like the San Pedro ceremonies in Peru, the ceremonies of the NAC are explicitly closed to outsiders.

That being said, any action taken to support peyote sustainability should naturally involve the people who hold it as a protected sacrament.

Legally speaking, the NAC was granted an exemption to use peyote on a religious basis after several decades of legal battles. Beyond the NAC, the sacrament remains illegal to use for those who are not members of federally recognized tribes. One cannot simply create their own version of a "native" church in an attempt to bypass this law and gain rights to use peyote. From some perspectives, this would be unethical exploitation of a hard-fought right to religious freedom reserved for sovereign nations.

RECIPROCITY IS NOT PHILANTHROPY

While researchers and cultural icons began exploring the use of mescaline for creativity and therapy last century, there was never any true reciprocity for the original cultures that shared this ancient medicine and healing tradition in the first place. Reciprocity is different from philanthropy in that it comes from a sense of mutuality, an understanding that "we are in this together," rather than from an ethic of charity.

Many people who benefit from psychedelics find themselves compelled to "give back" to the cultures that steward the medicine, including but not limited to the Amazonian tribes who steward ayahuasca or the Bwiti of Gabon, who steward iboga.

Considering that psychedelic therapy has its roots in the history of peyote and that the NAC is still fighting for sustainable access to their sacrament, it makes sense to direct some of that compulsion toward supporting local Native American tribes as well.

Support might look like getting involved with conservation efforts, advocating for the right of inmates from the NAC to access traditional spiritual ceremonies, or connecting with local Tribal organizations to donate any skills, finances, or labor that might be immediately useful.

But, to demonstrate reciprocity, people might also work on learning about the occupied land they live upon, the history of broken treaties in the United States, and the United Nations Nagoya Protocol — which is designed to create global frameworks for mutual benefit between indigenous people and the nations that utilize their sacred technologies.

PROPONENTS OF PSYCHEDELICS SHOULD SUPPORT PEYOTE SUSTAINABILITY

Peyote has a complex history in psychedelic research and therapy. The complexity arose in 1897 when the first psychedelic substance (mescaline) was isolated from peyote. At this time the U.S. government was waging war against Native American tribes and their ways of life. Combined with the fact that the psychedelic counterculture of the 1960s played a role in the over-harvesting and illegal poaching of this sacrament while never stepping in to help support the cultures it directly benefited from, there has long been an absence of mutual benefit or reciprocity.

Though researchers today are working to overcome this discrepancy and are currently studying the extent of long-term over-harvesting, the process is expensive, and the federal government does not intervene in the sustainability of Schedule 1 drugs facing extinction.

The Rio Grande Valley in Texas has been recognized for its natural beauty and peyote cultivation. The river that flows through this area provides ideal conditions when growing this sacred plant. In terms of environmental sustainability, it is essential to understand that peyote is critically threatened in Texas. Most all the land where the sacrament naturally grows is privately owned.

To grasp the concept of cultural sustainability, it's important to understand the full history.

The idea that chemists, doctors, and psychologists *discovered* psychedelic healthcare is a common misconception. Western anthropologists learned about psychedelic therapy by observing Native Americans' use of peyote, specifically members of the Comanche Tribe who had recently endured forced relocation to Oklahoma.

And yet, these facts alone do not tell the whole story. Gaining a deeply-rooted understanding of peyote's complex history might help demonstrate why both the environmental and cultural sustainability of peyote matter now more than ever.

SYNTHESIZED PSYCHEDELICS INSPIRED BY A PEYOTE CEREMONY

It's essential to know and understand the broader story behind the birth of the first *synthesized* psychedelic — otherwise, the truth will continue to be overlooked.

The roots of the NAC's sacred tipi ceremony emerged in the 19th century. During that time, Native American tribes were experiencing a horrific genocide and cultural erasure through forced relocations and the elimination of cultural rites, music, and ancestral lands. There are no words that may accurately convey the devastation felt by those who survived these events. And those who did survive these acts of genocide often found resilience in the one place the government would intervene — inside the tipi.

Before the NAC was established, the sacrament was either discovered by the tribes of the Southwest and Great Plains, or shared with them by guardians of the cactus, the Wixárika, or the Huichol as they are commonly referred to, who reside in the peyote cactus' natural habitat - Northern lands of present-day Mexico.

After 40 million bison were exterminated in an effort to starve the tribes, the massacre at Wounded Knee unfolded in 1890 and effectively marked a turning point in the U.S. war against Native Americans. Forcibly removed to reservations in Oklahoma and forced to live off limited Army rations, the peyote ceremony emerged as a therapeutic and unifying communal ritual for Native Americans.

In Oklahoma in 1896, James Mooney, an ethnographer working with the Smithsonian Institute, obtained a bag of the sacred mescaline-containing cacti from a Comanche elder named Quanah Parker. Mooney reported on the ceremony he witnessed, relaying in an article that "the Indians regard the mescal [cacti] as a panacea in medicine, a source of inspiration, and the key which opens to them all the glories of another world" (Jay, 2019).

Mooney's observations and the 50-pound bag of sacred cacti prompted Western researchers to take an interest in peyote's psychoactive effects (Abbott, 2019). One year later, in 1897, a German chemist named Arthur Hefter experimented with the sacred cactus and eventually isolated the psychoactive compound he called *meskalin* (Dinis-Oliveira, Pereira, & da Silva, 2019).

As Western researchers experimented further, developing mescaline tinctures and conducting self-experiments, the Native American tribes continued to face legal barriers (Rucker, Iliff, & Nutt, 2018). In 1912 a federal law was proposed to ban peyote use, but the bill did not clear the Senate because one Oklahoma Senator was persuaded by his constituents to reject it, and he, in turn, convinced his colleagues to pause on the measure.

After this, many anthropologists and leaders united with several Native American tribes to present evidence of peyote's sacramental use. In 1918 the Native American Church formed and fought several legal battles to protect access to their sacrament — which the government had tried to label as a controlled narcotic despite evidence of traditional use.

According to Western science, the rest of the story is history — psychiatric researcher Humphrey Osmond sat with author and philosopher Aldous Huxley on his first mescaline trip in 1953 (Tanne, 2004). Through a series of letters between the two, the word *psychedelic* — meaning "mind-manifesting" — was officially coined. Meanwhile, members of Native American tribes faced continued poverty and the violent abuse of boarding schools, not to mention continued legal battles to protect their right to use their sacrament. These battles continue today.

DRUG LAWS AND LAND DEVELOPMENT THREATEN PEYOTE

In the 1960s, the psychedelic movement took the world by storm. Enthusiasts were eager to try any substance that promised altered states of consciousness, and peyote was one of the most popular choices. Unfortunately, this led to over-harvesting and poaching of the cactus in the areas where it grows naturally.

The cactus grows extremely slowly, taking years to reach adulthood and decades to mature to a usable size. If appropriately harvested with roots undamaged, a cactus will produce medicine for decades, even hundreds of years — but poachers are not typically trained in traditional, sustainable harvesting practices. As a result, the peyote population has been severely depleted, and its survival is now at risk.

Peyote is now locally extinct from an ancient grove near Big Bend National Park, where poachers harvested the last cactus in 2019. In Mexico, the cactus is also facing sustainability issues resulting from drug tourism and illegal poaching. At this point, the NAC can hardly find enough medicine to meet the demands of its pan-tribal membership, estimated as of 2019 to include over 600,000 members.

Some see solutions to the sustainability concern in the form of greenhouses and mass production. For others, this is a stop-gap measure and an act of desperation, not a long-term solution for the

NAC and traditional wisdom holders. They believe that sustainable cultivation could occur — if the cactus were afforded the same level of protection as any other endangered plant.

But because peyote remains classified as a narcotic, landowners are hesitant to lease their private property for the purpose of peyote cultivation, especially when ranching is easier on insurance costs.

PEYOTE AS A PROTECTED SACRAMENT

There are two concepts related to the term sacrament that can be difficult to translate into the framework of Western scientific research: sacred and sovereign. These terms are occasionally confused with another term more common in the field of psychedelic therapy: cognitive liberty.

While sacred and sovereign convey notions of honor and responsibility, cognitive liberty suggests a more individualized interpretation of morality: that every individual has the right to think as they choose, and thus, the right to alter their consciousness in whatever style they wish — so long as they are not directly harming anyone but themselves in the process.

With this in mind, many people might feel compelled to cultivate peyote for their own use, believing it is an expression of personal liberty and a symbol of solidarity with the NAC and the Religious Freedom Restoration Act (Gatta, 2016).

However, this rationale might be premature and might be considered a form of scientific colonialism — especially if the peyote is used by providers or facilitators who work outside of the NAC. Just because the drug law is unnecessarily restrictive does not mean that peyote's religious protection is also redundant. And if there are to be laws that reconcile the legacy of colonization in the United States, what else might they look like, if not criminalization of offenders?

While some might find it difficult to imagine a reality where Native Americans are treated as sovereign nations, it is necessary for non-Native people to practice thinking in this way if they wish to support reciprocity for psychedelic healing.

As an exercise in cultural ethics, consider what the current state of psychedelic research might look like if Native American tribes had been approached ethically when mescaline was "discovered" back in 1897. In this alternative timeline, indigenous people, including the lineage holders in Mexico, would have been present and held as owners and benefactors of their own traditional ecological knowledge (TEK) at every step in the research process.

As Mooney reported after observing the peyote ceremony back in 1896, the knowledge and safe use of mescaline cacti were already clearly established in the oral history of indigenous cultures (Jay, 2019). If there were not already an effective protocol in place through ritual and ceremony, Western researchers would never have known the small cactus had any healing potential at all — and the entire story of psychedelic research would have taken on a very different timeline. Mescaline was not isolated from San Pedro until 1960, for example, and there is no reason to assume it would have been discovered any sooner (Ogunbodede, McCombs, Trout, Daley, & Terry, 2010).

Now, imagine if the right to access, grow, and sell peyote had also been protected for the past century. If this had been the case, it is more likely that peyote would not experience a sustainability crisis or face extinction as it does presently. And it is also likely that the economic health and security of many Native American tribes would be very different than it is today.

In terms of both environmental and cultural sustainability, it might be more important to support Native tribes working to develop their own development programs than to exercise one's idea of liberty in an effort toward solidarity. This is not to say that growing peyote is unethical (though it can be seen as disrespectful of the NAC), but rather to point out that it is not particularly helpful in addressing peyote sustainability concerns for the 600,000 members of the NAC. What would be more helpful is demonstrating reciprocity and solidarity for the cause in more direct ways. Offering financial support and donating time, skills, and labor towards lobbying and educational efforts are all important ways of showing up respectfully to support the indigenous peoples of the United States and Mexico, whose very cultures and ways of life are impacted by issues of peyote sustainability.

A FINAL THOUGHT

Peyote has been used for ceremonial and medicinal purposes by indigenous peoples in the Americas for millennia. Peyote grows mainly in northern Mexico and southern Texas and has been over-harvested and poached for the past 50 years. If this trend continues, peyote could become extinct in the wild. The Native American Church is the only federally recognized religion in the United States that uses peyote as a sacrament, and members of the Native American Church have been working to create an ethical, sustainable, and sovereign market for peyote. In order to avoid the tragedy of peyote becoming extinct, people and providers need to make commitments to work respectfully with Native American tribes to support an ethical, sustainable, and sovereign peyote market.

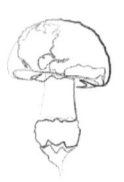

REFERENCES:

- Abbott, A. (2019). Altered minds: mescaline's complicated history. *Nature, 567(7757)*, 485-486. doi:10.1038/d41586-019-01571-
- Dinis-Oliveira, R. J., Pereira, C. L., & da Silva, D. D. (2019). Pharmacokinetic and Pharmacodynamic Aspects of Peyote and Mescaline: Clinical and Forensic Repercussions. *Curr Mol Pharmacol, 12*(3), 184-194. doi:10.2174/1874467211666181010154139
- Gatta, L. A. (2016). Conscience in the public square: The pivoting positions of the USCCB and ACLU around the Religious Freedom Restoration Act. *Linacre Q, 83*(4), 445-454. doi:10.1080/00243639.2016.1240007
- Jay, M. (2019). Mescaline : a global history of the first psychedelic. Retrieved from https://www.degruyter.com/isbn/9780300245080
- Ogunbodede, O., McCombs, D., Trout, K., Daley, P., & Terry, M. (2010). New mescaline concentrations from 14 taxa/cultivars of Echinopsis spp. (Cactaceae) ("San Pedro") and their relevance to shamanic practice. *J Ethnopharmacol, 131*(2), 356-362. doi:10.1016/j.jep.2010.07.021
- Rucker, J. J. H., Iliff, J., & Nutt, D. J. (2018). Psychiatry & the psychedelic drugs. Past, present & future. *Neuropharmacology, 142*, 200-218. doi:https://doi.org/10.1016/j.neuropharm.2017.12.040
- Tanne, J. H. (2004). Humphry Osmond. *BMJ : British Medical Journal, 328*(7441), 713-713. Retrieved from https://www.ncbi.nlm.nih.gov/pmc/articles/PMC381240/

THIRTY
PEYOTE LEGALITY AND RELIGIOUS FREEDOM FOR SETTLERS
ALICE DE WITT

Psychedelics have been used for religious and spiritual purposes throughout history. In many cultures, they are seen as a sacred medicine that can facilitate deep personal transformation. In recent years, there has been a growing interest in the use of psychedelics for spiritual and religious purposes. Some argue that any psychedelic that can facilitate mystical experiences should be legal for religious use. While this argument may be intuitive and rational, it lacks some social and historical context. This chapter hopes to offer a little support in that regard, especially as it pertains to the peyote cactus.

Let's be clear from the get-go: as you read about in the previous chapter, peyote is a naturally occurring but critically threatened sacramental cactus that produces mescaline, the same psychoactive compound found in San Pedro cactus. This small yet powerful plant played an important role during The Psychedelic Renaissance; it is the compound that inspired the term "psychedelic."

From today's (slightly) more progressive standpoint, the idea that peyote should be protected as part of our right to religious freedom may seem both intuitive and logical. But this was not always the case, and in fact, Native Americans were persecuted and killed for using peyote in ceremonies, which settlers could only conceive of as an evil narcotic rather than as the healing medicine and sacrament it was known to be among those who practice Peyotism faith of the Native American Church (NAC).

Before we dive into the details of the legal history of peyote, let's establish some groundwork around settler relationships.

POLICY DISCUSSIONS FROM THE HEART

Settlers who engaged in discussions about decolonization and Native American genocide often experience unprocessed feelings of guilt, shame, or righteousness. These emotions are valid but should be worked through before engaging with policy-related issues concerning peyote use. Working our way through this gives us more insight into who we are and where we come from, leaving us better equipped to have a conversation about settler colonialism and the impact of peyote laws on religious freedom. Without having some awareness of our own roots or grounding in our own sense of place, we can run into problems of romanticization and tokenizing of indigenous cultures, relying on media portrayals or tropes. For example, many falsely assume that Native Americans only live on reservations in tipis, but over three-quarters live outside of reservations in cities throughout what is now called the United States.

This brief exercise can be helpful when considering the use of any sacred plant medicine. However, it is especially important for the United States, where peyote is critically threatened, and religious freedom is still in question.

WHERE ARE YOU?

Before we jump into the legal history of peyote in the United States, take a minute to visit native-land.ca. Figure out quickly where you are and what land you're living on. Note the original stewards and the languages spoken and do a little research to see the status of the tribe currently. Are some fully recognized tribes? Or are they unrecognized? Where is the local Tribal Authority located? If you have an extra minute, look up where your parents and grandparents lived in the United States (if this applies), and do the same.

The point of this exercise is to remind us that we walk and live on stolen land. The United States is a colonial nation that has yet to reconcile its history of conquest, and this history is interwoven with past and current peyote policy discussions.

FEDERAL LEGISLATION THAT IMPACTED PEYOTE USE

Before peyote was exempted from the Controlled Substances Act in 1970, there were several pieces of legislation detailing the rights of Native Americans and religious sacraments and ceremonies.

This list is not exhaustive, but we hope it is a start:

The Bureau of Indian Affairs is Established in 1824

Native peoples in the United States have a long and complicated history with the federal government. Beginning in 1806, Congress established the Office of Indian Trade, which was tasked with regulating trade and land transactions involving Native peoples. The office was housed within the War Department, and traders were licensed to operate within Native territories. In 1924, the office became the Bureau of Indian Affairs, and Native leaders were given directorial positions within the department. These leaders were tasked with maintaining relations with Tribes and overseeing federal policies. Throughout its evolution, the Bureau of Indian Affairs has played a significant role in the lives of Native peoples in the United States.

The 1830 Indian Removal Act
In 1829, a gold rush emerged in Georgia, driving up land speculation and attracting settlers. After Southern states attempted to draft their laws to extinguish land titles among Native Americans, President Andrew Johnson signed the Indian Removal Act. In an act of genocide, this measure funded the forced relocation of several Native American Tribes from their ancestral lands in the Southeast to territories west of the Mississippi. Some organizers and missionaries protested the act. It was heavily debated in Congress before ultimately passing, with 28 in favor and 19 opposed. The "forced removal" process lasted over a decade and would go on to be known in U.S. history as the Trail of Tears.
Once on Indian Territory land, the Tribes were told they would be left alone to self-rule, but this was not the case. It was through intertribal relationships that Peyotism emerged and was shared. There were similarly forced migrations of indigenous populations in the North, with several cases related to land captures and broken treaties.

The Religious Crimes Code of 1883
The Code of Indian Offenses was passed by the United States Congress in 1866 as a way to establish law and order among Native American tribes. The main goal of the code was to "civilize" Native Americans and force them to assimilate into white society. Under the code, a Court of Indian Offenses was established, which had the power to interfere with criminal justice in sovereign Native nations. This led to a lot of abuse and mistreatment of Native Americans, as the government oftentimes used force to enforce the laws.

As a result, many Native Americans lost their culture and way of life. The Code of Indian Offenses was an act of cultural genocide that caused immense harm to Native American communities.

Punishable offenses included gathering together, dancing, singing, using drums, giving gifts, carrying ceremonial items, and practicing any cultural custom that was seen as "uncivilized." Settlers even targeted the Potlatch ceremony common to many tribes of the Pacific Northwest. The word "potluck" comes from the traditional potlatch that remained illegal in Canada until 1951, but then, the ritual practice of resource sharing was seen as detrimental to the nation's character. Peyote ceremonies were not permitted.

The Dawes Act of 1887

In continued efforts toward assimilation, the United States government initiated a measure to break up remaining Tribal territories into individual parcels that Native Americans were expected to use for farming and agriculture, never mind that farming was not practical on the lands provided. The Army and hunters drove the bison to near extinction to make room for cattle ranching and simultaneously tried to make some Tribes dependent upon the settlers for food and resources. In total, the United States government claimed another two-thirds of the remaining Sovereign land base through legislation that fractured families and tribal leadership.

If Native Americans complied, the U.S. would grant citizenship rights. If they did not, the U.S. would sell the allotments of tribal land to non-Native citizens at a fraction of the cost. The act was another effort at assimilation, forcing European American agricultural practices onto Native American tribes. This Act also formed the basis for the use of "blood-quantum" (aka the "amount" or ratio of Native American "blood" as defined through genealogy) as a means of establishing federally recognized tribal membership, a necessary precursor for gaining rights and access to programs and religious protections for sacramental peyote.

The Indian Reorganization Act of 1934

At the turn of the century, the United States began to address drug laws internationally and nationally. The Pure Food and Drug Act was passed in 1906, paving the way for the Harrison Act of 1914, which would threaten the traditional use of peyote and peyote ceremony. Up until this point, Peyotism was practiced in the safety and isolation of the tipi, the one place where Federal interference seemed to stall. But settlers consistently saw peyote as a narcotic rather than the sacrament it is. As early as 1893, Parke-Davis, a pharmaceutical company in Detroit, sold peyote tincture as a stimulant. Researchers were using peyote in human trials to try and mimic schizophrenia as early as 1913.

In 1928, the federal government commissioned the Meriam Report to investigate the state of health on the reservations. Amidst reservation schooling and the intergenerational effects of genocide, the report made clear that Congress had failed to protect the well-being of Native American Tribes on reservations. Part of President Roosevelt's New Deal was the American Indian New Deal, whose main goal was to reverse the impact of the Dawes Act. As part of this effort, John Collier issued a mandate that no "interference with Indian religious life or ceremonial expression will hereafter be tolerated. The cultural liberty of Indians is in all respects to be considered equal to that of any non-Indian group."

The Indian Civil Rights Act of 1968 and Peyote Exemption to the CSA in 1970

The American Indian Movement was founded in 1968 in response to the continued mistreatment of Native Americans by settlers and the U.S. government. Even after the U.S. government had put into place various legal protections for Native Americans, settlers continued to commit acts of racism and harassment against them. The AIM was deeply involved in activism and advocacy for civil rights and religious protections for Native Americans. Thanks in part to the efforts of the AIM, Native Americans now have more legal protections and are better able to preserve their culture and way of life.

AIM engaged in public actions to draw awareness to the realities of settler injustice against Native Americans, especially in response to further assimilation measures. And as the Controlled Substances Act moved forward under Nixon, Native American advocates and a handful of allies in Congress effectively argued for the exclusion of peyote from Schedule 1 for NAC ceremonial use. However, the full extent of the Bill of Rights, including freedom of religion, was not yet guaranteed under this act.

The American Indian Religious Freedom Act of 1978

Under President Jimmy Carter, Congress finally enacted legislation to explicitly extend the full rights of religious freedom to Native Americans. Known as AIRFA, these protections extended to ceremonies, access to sacred sites, and ritual elements collected from sacred animals being held in every state, regardless of existing state laws. However, without a penalty provision, the act lacked any teeth or power of enforcement in the event states ignored the request and allowed construction on top of a sacred site, mining of a sacred mountain, logging in sacred forests, or dams on sacred rivers.

Lacking any sense of reciprocity, some states began interpreting AIRFA in ways that caused further harm to Native

American tribes, including denying the use of peyote for religious purposes.

The Religious Freedom Restoration Act of 1993 and Religious Land Use of Institutionalized Persons Act of 2000

In the early 1980s, a number of federal courts began re-interpreting the Religious Freedom Act, suggesting that the law did not actually protect the use of peyote, a Schedule I controlled substance. This interpretation was based on the fact that peyote is illegal under federal and state law, and therefore its use could not be considered "religious." However, a handful of court cases challenged this interpretation, and the U.S. Supreme Court made it abundantly clear that peyote use was protected under the Religious Freedom Act. In doing so, the Court held that courts must use "strict scrutiny" when interpreting the 1st Amendment, which guarantees the free exercise of religion.

A 1997 case in Texas challenged the ruling, as a Catholic church sued the city for rejecting a proposal to expand their premises on the grounds that zoning ordinances would also fall under this "strict scrutiny" of religious freedom interpretation. In response, several states ended up establishing their own versions of the religious freedom act, shifting the decision-making power around enforcement of religious freedom laws around peyote back to the state. Often called "mini-RFRAs," these measures vary and are evolving, but most do not prioritize conversations with people who practice Peyotism.

After RFRA was struck down in 1997, Congress responded with the Religious Land Use of Institutionalized Persons Act in 2000, guaranteeing that incarcerated individuals would still be granted religious freedom when in prison. This has permitted the use of the Sweat Lodge ceremony among Native

American inmates in some prisons, which has demonstrated benefits in rehabilitation.

SUPPORTING NATIVE AMERICAN SOVEREIGNTY BY SUPPORTING RELIGIOUS FREEDOM FOR ENTHEOGENS

This chapter sought to offer a primer on some important legal cases and decisions that have impacted both peyote law and religious freedom in the United States. Many people who experience the spiritual benefits of psychedelic medicines argue that these experiences should be protected under the Religious Freedom Act and often point to peyote as an example to justify their argument.

But as we have hopefully demonstrated in this brief, one-sided review of legislation from a settler perspective, the context of these arguments could benefit from more intentional collaboration and dialogue between all those who are impacted by prohibitive and oppressive laws. Collaboration happens in relationships, and relationships need to be consensual and reciprocal if they are to be sustainable. And in this regard, psychedelic healthcare access could be a bridge of understanding that opens up further awareness of the rights and realities of Native American tribes.

For more information, visit the Native American Rights Fund and the National Congress of American Indians. If you are interested in learning more about supporting Sovereignty, take note of the Sorgorea Te' Land Trust and the Shuumi Land Tax effort, and the Land Back Movement.

PART NINE
IBOGAINE

"Not why the addiction but why the pain."

Dr. Gabor Maté

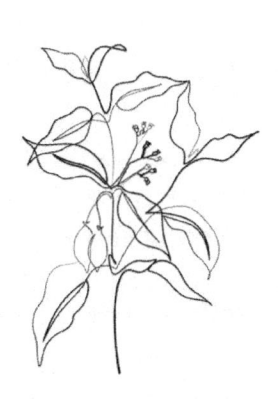

THIRTY-ONE
A BEGINNER'S GUIDE TO IBOGAINE
KATIE STONE, MA

MEDICALLY REVIEWED BY DR. BENJAMIN MALCOLM, PHARMD, MPH, BCPP

Ibogaine is a psychoactive indole alkaloid found in several species of plants. The most well-known is *Tabernanthe iboga*, a slow-growing perennial shrub from western Africa. *Tabernanthe iboga*, commonly called Iboga, is only native to three nations. It is most abundant in Gabon but also in parts of the Democratic Republic of the Congo (DRC) and Cameroon. The compound is also naturally occurring in several other plants, including *Voacanga africana* and *Tabernaemontana undulata*.

In the 1960s, ibogaine was brought to the Western world's attention when it was found to have the ability to eliminate opioid withdrawals in persons physically dependent on opioids. Since then, ibogaine has continued to be used in the treatment of opioid addiction. Ibogaine may also have the potential to treat diseases of the nervous system, such as Parkinson's disease, but until clinical trials are fully permitted, the full healing potential of ibogaine is unknown and unverified (Bhat et al., 2021). Despite its promising potential, ibogaine remains a controversial substance due to its hallucinogenic properties. However, as more research is conducted on ibogaine's therapeutic potential, it is possible that this substance will one day be accepted as a viable treatment for a variety of conditions.

There are serious and unique risks associated with ibogaine compared to other psychedelics, and it is not generally considered safe — unless one has had the proper medical evaluations to confirm their health status. And even then, death can occur (Noller, Frampton, & Yazar-Klosinski, 2018). Some health conditions and medications are contraindicated and have potentially lethal risks. It is vital to find ibogaine facilitators who are well-trained and experienced and clinics that conduct proper medical screenings. But because ibogaine therapy is unregulated, it is up to the patient to advocate for their wellbeing.

IBOGAINE'S LEGAL STATUS

Ibogaine is a Schedule 1 drug in the United States and has been listed as illegal since the 1970 Controlled Substances Act. It is also illegal in nine countries in the European Union and is mostly unregulated everywhere else (being neither legal nor illegal). In Brazil, New Zealand, and South Africa, ibogaine is a regulated pharmaceutical that physicians can prescribe.

The primary source of ibogaine is derived from iboga, a protected species in Gabon, a West African nation that banned all ibogaine exports in 2019. Since the United Nations Nagoya Protocol and a 2000 declaration that designated iboga a "national cultural heritage" and "strategic reserve to be protected from illegal exploitation," thus affording additional legal protections to this cultural sacrament.

LEGAL IBOGAINE CLINICS

It is vital to find an ibogaine clinic that conducts a full medical screening because ibogaine can be highly toxic.

Ibogaine treatment centers are available across the world, mostly in accordance with the global patchwork quilt created by varying legality across jurisdictions. Adequate medical screening, as well as monitoring and available care in the event of medical emergencies, are important components of safe use.

Integration is an important part of the ibogaine experience. Immediately after the main effects of the medicine have worn off, it is common for persons to feel a range of emotions, including confusion and disorientation. For this reason, it is important to have access to support during this time. Some ibogaine treatment centers may offer extended recovery support, while others may encourage persons to find these services independently. However, working with a provider or ibogaine integration counselor - either near you or remotely - can help to ensure long-term success. These professionals can provide guidance and support during the early stages of integration, helping you to make sustainable behavior changes. In addition, they can offer ongoing assistance as you continue to navigate the challenges and opportunities of life after ibogaine treatment.

PHARMACOLOGY OF IBOGAINE

Ibogaine's impacts and toxicity are not fully understood, but it has a unique mechanism of action (Glue et al., 2015). The cardiac toxicity possible with ibogaine also sets it apart from other psychedelics. While ibogaine appears anti-addictive for many drugs that lead to substance use disorders, it can actually block or greatly diminish the acute withdrawal effects of opioids, making it particularly well suited for treating opioid use disorder (Malcolm, Polanco, & Barsuglia, 2018).

Ibogaine significantly impacts the heart's electrical conduction system, which can lead to lowered heart rates and arrhythmias. This can be fatal and is the primary reason why a medical screening with an electrocardiogram (EKG) reading that includes the QTc Interval reading is necessary. Cardiac arrest can occur in the days following ibogaine use, and centers should not discharge people for at least 72 hours after treatment.

Because of its broad physiological effects, many medications are dangerous to mix with ibogaine (Litjens & Brunt, 2016). Heart medications, psychiatric medications, and medications that prolong QTc intervals or inhibit liver enzymes can all be dangerous.

Currently, the doses of ibogaine used for opioid dependencies in published literature have ranged from 8-20mg/kg (Mash, Duque, Page, & Allen-Ferdinand, 2018). Full doses used to treat serious addictions are sometimes referred to as 'flood' doses. Several deaths have occurred at around 30mg/kg (Alper, Stajić, & Gill, 2012; Noller et al., 2018). However, doses as low as 4mg/kg have resulted in death in persons using contraindicated drugs or with pre-existing cardiovascular disease (Alper et al., 2012).

Ibogaine interacts across multiple neurotransmitter systems (Coleman et al., 2019). It is active on sigma-2 and multiple opioid receptor sites. It also interacts with acetylcholine, dopamine, and serotonin systems. Ibogaine is an antagonist at the NMDA glutamate receptor. Additionally, noribogaine appears to further engage with mu and kappa opioid receptors after it's metabolized in the body from its source molecule, ibogaine.

Unique among psychedelics, one study found ibogaine stimulates and modulates the release of a protein known as GDNF (glial cell line-derived neurotrophic factor) (Ly et al., 2018). GDNF plays a unique role in maintaining the health of dopamine receptors (Carnicella & Ron, 2009). Ibogaine also modulates the neurological systems that release BDNF (brain-derived neurotrophic factor), a protein that supports nerve cells' survival and growth (Litjens & Brunt, 2016).

RISKS ASSOCIATED WITH IBOGAINE USE

There are several risks of using ibogaine associated with its psychedelic effects or properties. For this reason, attention to set and setting is important to reduce psychological risks. Those with a history of mania or psychosis should not use ibogaine as it may create more problems than solutions. During ibogaine therapy, electrolyte imbalances can be dangerous with any size dose.

There have been at least 27 reported deaths from ibogaine treatment, due to the unregulated nature of the ibogaine industry, many deaths go unreported (Litjens & Brunt, 2016). Some estimates place the average death rate at 1 in 300. Heart complications are a severe risk because ibogaine extends the QT interval and causes lowered blood pressure and heart rates. Proper medical pre-screening and expert supervision can help minimize this risk and improve the safety of ibogaine therapies. Risks should always be considered alongside the possible benefits.

PRE-EXISTING HEALTH CONDITIONS AND MEDICATION RISKS OF IBOGAINE

Because of its broad physiological effects, many medications are dangerous to mix with ibogaine. Heart medications, psychiatric medications, long-acting opioid medications (i.e., methadone, buprenorphine, oxycontin), medications that prolong QTc intervals, inhibit CYP2D6 liver enzymes, and others can all be dangerous. Some contraindicated medications include beta-blockers, stimulants, and fluoxetine.

Other conditions such as non-drug-induced seizure disorders such as epilepsy, respiratory conditions, some severe gastrointestinal conditions, liver impairment, as well as some psychiatric conditions may exclude someone from ibogaine treatment. Individuals diagnosed with morbid obesity may also be at greater risk for adverse events.

People with hepatitis C, HIV, blood pressure problems (or taking blood pressure medication), and a history of alcoholism should be screened thoroughly by an experienced facilitator.

MENTAL HEALTH RISKS ASSOCIATED WITH IBOGAINE

Because of the risks of complications, the simplest thing one can do to reduce risk is never to use ibogaine alone or outside the supervision of a skilled provider. Using ibogaine may reveal underlying mental health conditions, and there are also psychological risks to consider beyond the previously mentioned physical risks.

Individuals diagnosed with schizophrenia or with a history of psychosis may be at increased risk for exacerbated symptoms of their diagnoses when taking ibogaine. Mental health diagnoses and behavioral patterns can often help providers determine who makes a safe ibogaine therapy candidate. People who have been hospitalized for bipolar disorder, borderline personality disorder, depersonalization, psychosis, or mania should share these experiences with their providers to determine the best course of action.

THE HISTORY OF IBOGAINE

In its original context, iboga supports members of Bwiti through rites and rituals that originate in a pre-colonial era.

The iboga plant is the sacred sacrament of the Bwiti spiritual discipline, one of three officially recognized religions in Gabon.

Roughly translated, *bwiti* means *ancestor*, and the iboga plant serves as the sacrament that opens the door to the spirit world.

The mystical experiences elicited by iboga are considered essential components for health, healing, and culture. In small doses, the iboga plant was used to improve hunting skills. In larger doses, it is used to connect with the ancestors and initiate youth into their tribal culture and family.

Iboga is often found along elephant trails. The animals eat the fruit and spread the seeds, and there are stories of elephants digging up roots and acting erratically. According to folklore, a woman ate a porcupine and experienced incredible visions and a shamanic journey into the root of herself and spirit — she found out afterward that the porcupine had been eating iboga root and shared this wisdom with the village.

Modern rituals today are often infused with elements from other religions (such as Christianity). Ancestors and animism are integral elements of Bwiti, and iboga is used to facilitate healing and initiate one into a spiritual lineage through rites of passage.

French colonists observed the rituals and brought iboga back to Europe, where ibogaine was isolated and manufactured as *Lambarène*. Instead of a religious sacrament, ibogaine was now a "neuromuscular stimulant" pressed into a 200 mg tablet that held 8 mg of ibogaine hydrochloride said to treat "fatigue, depression, and recovery from infectious disease" (Brown & Alper, 2018).

In the 1960s, ibogaine emerged as a folk remedy for addiction before being labeled a Schedule 1 drug under the 1970 Controlled Substances Act. While the U.S. began the War on Drugs, Chilean psychiatrist Claudio Naranjo used ibogaine alongside psychotherapy, and Howard Lotsof pioneered ibogaine therapy in New York City among fellow heroin users experiencing addiction.

By the 1980s, ibogaine was patented as an interrupter of narcotic addiction, and by the 1990s, recovery advocate Eric Taub had catalyzed the underground ibogaine movement in the United States to support people who experience substance dependencies. It was from this underground protocol, often taking place in hotel rooms, that centers with medical staff and new safety protocols started emerging in Mexico and Central America — where drug scheduling was less stringent.

Since then, several studies have demonstrated the impact ibogaine has on opioid self-administration and withdrawal (Malcolm et al., 2018). Alcohol and cocaine consumption has also been researched, albeit less thoroughly (Cappendijk & Dzoljic, 1993; He et al., 2005). Researchers today explore ibogaine analogs that operate on the same receptors without psychoactive side effects and the risks of physical harm associated with ibogaine.

The current opioid epidemic and subsequent national public health emergency that opioid addiction has created in the US has brought conversations about ibogaine back to the forefront, and some states or cities have made moves to decriminalize ibogaine or make it available for the treatment of opioid addiction.

IS USING IBOGAINE ETHICAL?

There are unique ethical concerns around the risks of using ibogaine and also around biopiracy and threats to the iboga shrub and its sustainability and natural habitat.

People suffering from life-threatening dependencies may look to iboga as a substitute for addiction treatment. If unable to access the concentrated ibogaine HCl used at clinics, people may seek the alternative iboga root bark to try and alleviate symptoms.

For some practitioners, separating ibogaine from the Bwiti ritual is unethical and dangerous — because the ritual can help support the mystical therapeutic experiences that inspire long-term behavior change. Bwiti members claim that their music, made up of jaw harps and stringed instruments, may function in ceremony to help regulate the heart rate and nervous system, although there are no clinical trials that have tested this idea.

Traditional ceremony is not without risk, and deaths have been reported at clinics that incorporate Bwiti ritual but lack experience in managing Western pharmaceuticals. Recognizing that most Westerners who seek out ibogaine are doing so to address ill health, it is important that participants communicate the extent of their health status to their providers and retreat centers, seek medical supervision when appropriate, and arrive prepared with travel medical insurance in the event of an emergency. Likewise, it is imperative for providers to approach ibogaine with a clear understanding of risks and to spare no effort in medical screening, monitoring, and access to emergency care.

The area where iboga grows naturally is also impacted by elephant poaching, and elephant poachers will often harvest and sell iboga illegally online to unsuspecting consumers. Widespread Western use has resulted in the illegal poaching and over-harvesting of sacred iboga, directly impacting the local communities who rely on this medicine.

As the ethical concerns around iboga sustainability are addressed, some providers and clinics commit to only using the more sustainably cultivated ibogaine HCl derived from *Voacanga africana*. Supporting clinics that demonstrate this commitment is probably the most sustainable way to work with ibogaine therapy for addiction.

HEALING POTENTIAL OF IBOGAINE

Preclinical trials suggest ibogaine might support long-term positive psychological outcomes, and ibogaine might be the most effective opiate detox aid (Brown & Alper, 2018). Remission rates range from 75% in a small one-year observational study to 50% at a one-month follow-up in another study (Noller et al., 2018). It should be noted these studies lack control groups and lost many participants to follow-up, which could conceivably skew perceptions of favorable outcomes.

Ibogaine's potential for treating addiction is the most well-known but is not the only reported therapeutic benefit of ibogaine. Anecdotal reports reveal many benefits from using ibogaine, or its root plant, iboga. But until research is conducted, the healing potential of ibogaine will continue to be poorly understood.

Drawing similarities from other psychedelic compounds that interact on similar receptors, one might be able to imagine the potential for ibogaine to elicit the same sort of mystical experiences known to have a lasting impact. And considering that the Bwiti use iboga as a sacrament, one might gather that there is a spiritual element to ibogaine's healing potential. However, only a few studies currently investigate the subjective experiences of healing among people who use ibogaine (Brown, Noller, & Denenberg, 2019; Heink, Katsikas, & Lange-Altman, 2017; Schenberg et al., 2017).

WHAT TO EXPECT FROM AN IBOGAINE TRIP

Ibogaine is neither a gentle psychedelic on the mind nor the body. It is not known to be euphoric or pleasant in its effects. It is technically an oneiric rather than a hallucinogen and creates a lucid dream-like state that can last for 24 hours or longer.

The ibogaine experience is typically very intense and often includes visions. One may be faced with the truth of their traumas while undergoing an uncomfortable or risky physical transformation. Some participants don't have any visual hallucinations but instead hear auditory ones. Ideally, you'll find yourself safe enough during your trip so as not distracted by external factors which could jeopardize this powerful visionary journey.

People receiving therapy at an ibogaine treatment center will undergo a medical evaluation during intake. In an ideal setting, the patient will undergo a test dose followed by an EKG test, followed by days of observation to guarantee there are no adverse reactions — but this is a rare practice as ibogaine treatment centers often only book people for a handful of days. If you are interested in ibogaine treatment, take your time to find a provider who works safely.

An ibogaine treatment at a complete or flood dose may last more than 24 hours, with peak experiences beginning within the first three hours. The first half of the experience leaves people wanting to lie down. Most report a range of sensations from rushing energy, nausea, increased heart rate, irregular breathing rate, loss of coordination, and dizziness. Dizziness and feeling off-balance (ataxia), as well as experiencing dry mouth and tremors is also common. During the dream state, people report experiencing memories, insights, and visions; some people have profound epiphanies during this time.

Post-experience effects can last for several days, an ideal time for reflection and integration. Some people report revitalized energy; others may prefer to rest as the second-day post-treatment is said to be especially difficult as the brain's neurotransmitters re-stabilize. Noribogaine, ibogaine's metabolite, stays active in the body for days after ibogaine administration. From a safety perspective, it is important to stay away from other substances during this time.

PREPARING FOR AN IBOGAINE EXPERIENCE

Preparations for an ibogaine trip will begin with a medical evaluation and evolve according to the participants' needs. People should be preparing for ibogaine with the help of an experienced and qualified practitioner.

Preparations can also take on a spiritual tone, with participants engaging in mindfulness practices like journaling, intention setting, and ritual to nurture the psyche toward a transformative or transpersonal state. Working with a practitioner in the months following an ibogaine treatment will help people integrate their insights and visionary experiences into something meaningful in their lives.

HOW TO CHOOSE AN IBOGAINE TREATMENT CENTER

As a potentially lethal psychedelic, ibogaine is not one to take lightly. Working with qualified and experienced professionals can help lessen the risk of death and harm. Avoid ibogaine treatment centers that forget to make clear the risks associated with this psychedelic and look for any red flags that might lead to dangerous situations.

A treatment center should be asking for blood work and EKGs and should have a robust and well-practiced emergency plan ready to go. Trained medical professionals should be on hand, and the nearest emergency room should be known to everyone on the team. A total intake of drug use, medications, supplements, and health history should be assessed as well. If all these conditions are not present, then look for another ibogaine treatment center.

Online reviews can be misleading, so it is a good idea to find people who have attended an ibogaine treatment center and ask for honest feedback. Also, ask the center to provide reviews and references. Researching the center's background and management can also reveal any hidden scandals or deaths that do not turn up on a standard search.

Looking for ibogaine treatment centers connected to communities that offer vetted referrals can help people make informed decisions and networks of ibogaine providers that make commitments toward ethical practice. While the world of ibogaine therapy is rapidly evolving, it will be critical to keep safety the top priority for all involved.

Ibogaine offers unique therapeutic potential on both a molecular and spiritual level — most significantly in relation to opioid dependencies. It has been traditionally used for Bwiti ceremonies but can also be found at medical clinics or retreat centers that aim to blend allopathic medicine with the traditional use of this powerful plant extract. Medical screening and monitoring should always be used to maintain the highest level of safety. The risks of ibogaine are considerable yet can be minimized with clear communication, proper medical screening, and access to emergency care.

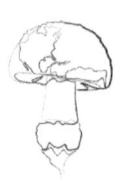

REFERENCES:

- Alper, K. R., Stajić, M., & Gill, J. R. (2012). Fatalities temporally associated with the ingestion of ibogaine. *J Forensic Sci, 57*(2), 398-412. doi:10.1111/j.1556-4029.2011.02008.x
- Brown, T. K., & Alper, K. (2018). Treatment of opioid use disorder with ibogaine: detoxification and drug use outcomes. *Am J Drug Alcohol Abuse, 44*(1), 24-36. doi:10.1080/00952990.2017.1320802
- Brown, T. K., Noller, G. E., & Denenberg, J. O. (2019). Ibogaine and Subjective Experience: Transformative States and Psychopharmacotherapy in the Treatment of Opioid Use Disorder. *J Psychoactive Drugs, 51*(2), 155-165. doi:10.1080/02791072.2019.1598603

- Cappendijk, S. L., & Dzoljic, M. R. (1993). Inhibitory effects of ibogaine on cocaine self-administration in rats. *Eur J Pharmacol, 241*(2-3), 261-265. doi:10.1016/0014-2999(93)90212-z
- Carnicella, S., & Ron, D. (2009). GDNF--a potential target to treat addiction. *Pharmacology & therapeutics, 122*(1), 9-18. doi:10.1016/j.pharmthera.2008.12.001
- Coleman, J. A., Yang, D., Zhao, Z., Wen, P. C., Yoshioka, C., Tajkhorshid, E., & Gouaux, E. (2019). Serotonin transporter-ibogaine complexes illuminate mechanisms of inhibition and transport. *Nature, 569*(7754), 141-145. doi:10.1038/s41586-019-1135-1
- Glue, P., Winter, H., Garbe, K., Jakobi, H., Lyudin, A., Lenagh-Glue, Z., & Hung, C. T. (2015). Influence of CYP2D6 activity on the pharmacokinetics and pharmacodynamics of a single 20 mg dose of ibogaine in healthy volunteers. *The Journal of Clinical Pharmacology, 55*(6), 680-687. doi:https://doi.org/10.1002/jcph.471
- He, D. Y., McGough, N. N., Ravindranathan, A., Jeanblanc, J., Logrip, M. L., Phamluong, K., . . . Ron, D. (2005). Glial cell line-derived neurotrophic factor mediates the desirable actions of the anti-addiction drug ibogaine against alcohol consumption. *J Neurosci, 25*(3), 619-628. doi:10.1523/jneurosci.3959-04.2005
- Heink, A., Katsikas, S., & Lange-Altman, T. (2017). Examination of the Phenomenology of the Ibogaine Treatment Experience: Role of Altered States of Consciousness and Psychedelic Experiences. *J Psychoactive Drugs, 49*(3), 201-208. doi:10.1080/02791072.2017.1290855
- Litjens, R. P., & Brunt, T. M. (2016). How toxic is ibogaine? *Clin Toxicol (Phila), 54*(4), 297-302. doi:10.3109/15563650.2016.1138226

- Ly, C., Greb, A. C., Cameron, L. P., Wong, J. M., Barragan, E. V., Wilson, P. C., . . . Olson, D. E. (2018). Psychedelics Promote Structural and Functional Neural Plasticity. *Cell reports, 23*(11), 3170-3182. doi:10.1016/j.celrep.2018.05.022
- Malcolm, B. J., Polanco, M., & Barsuglia, J. P. (2018). Changes in Withdrawal and Craving Scores in Participants Undergoing Opioid Detoxification Utilizing Ibogaine. *J Psychoactive Drugs, 50*(3), 256-265. doi:10.1080/02791072.2018.1447175
- Mash, D. C., Duque, L., Page, B., & Allen-Ferdinand, K. (2018). Ibogaine Detoxification Transitions Opioid and Cocaine Abusers Between Dependence and Abstinence: Clinical Observations and Treatment Outcomes. *Frontiers in pharmacology, 9*, 529-529. doi:10.3389/fphar.2018.00529
- Noller, G. E., Frampton, C. M., & Yazar-Klosinski, B. (2018). Ibogaine treatment outcomes for opioid dependence from a twelve-month follow-up observational study. *Am J Drug Alcohol Abuse, 44*(1), 37-46. doi:10.1080/00952990.2017.1310218
- Schenberg, E., Comis, M. A., Alexandre, J., Tófoli, L. F., Chaves, B., & Silveira, D. (2017). A phenomenological analysis of the subjective experience elicited by ibogaine in the context of a drug dependence treatment. *Journal of Psychedelic Studies, 1*, 1-10. doi:10.1556/2054.01.2017.007

THIRTY-TWO
IBOGAINE FOR SUBSTANCE DEPENDENCY
SHEA PRUEGER AND KATIE STONE, MA

MEDICALLY REVIEWED BY DR. BENJAMIN MALCOLM, PHARMD, MPH, BCPP

Iboga is a powerful psychoactive substance that has been used for millennia by the pygmy people of equatorial West Africa. Presently, iboga use is concentrated in the Bwiti tribes of Gabon. Iboga is a part of everyday life in Gabon, used to aid wakefulness on long hunting excursions or to uplift mood at celebrations, it is also used for initiation rites and ceremonial rituals. Ibogaine, an indole alkaloid derived from the root bark (also referred to as iboga) of the equatorial West African perennial shrub *Tabernanthe iboga*, which is part of the Apocynaceae family and has gained popularity as a treatment for substance dependency. It is most known for its ability to eliminate withdrawals from opiates and also for its intense, long, rapid-eye-movement-induced visionary journey. *Beyond* its documented ability to eliminate opioid withdrawals, it is reportedly profound at healing substance use disorders (SUD), commonly referred to as addiction. Although there is still much to learn about the potential benefits of ibogaine, it shows promise as a treatment for substance dependencies.

There are many self-reports and observational studies of withdrawal symptoms from short-acting opiates (SAOs) such as heroin being completely eliminated within one to two hours of ibogaine ingestion. Aside from eliminating withdrawal symptoms in opioid-dependent people, ibogaine also reduces substance cravings, potentially lowering the risk of continued drug use in individuals with dependencies on narcotics. In recent years, peer-reviewed journals have highlighted the benefits of using ibogaine to treat dependencies to stimulants such as cocaine and methamphetamine, opioids, nicotine, and alcohol. Anecdotally, forums on the internet dedicated to discussing ibogaine claim it may work for other compulsive behaviors.

The World Health Organization (WHO) reports that 35 million people have a SUD, yet long-term treatment solutions are lacking. Ibogaine is an alternative treatment that has helped many, and the ones it has helped often become inspired by the possibility of it helping others.

It is important to remember that ibogaine alone is not a cure or 'magic bullet' for addiction and needs to be paired with proactive solutions for learning healthy coping mechanisms for long-term success. This can include integrating the ibogaine experience, engaging with addiction recovery and support therapies or programs, creating new behavioral patterns, addressing trauma, and other lifestyle changes that maintain or improve health.

RESEARCH ON IBOGAINE

Research regarding ibogaine pales compared to other psychedelics such as psilocybin and ketamine, possibly due to the fatalities associated with ibogaine and its perception of being very dangerous and subjectively unpleasant. Still, we do have some research, and it's promising.

Ibogaine and noribogaine have demonstrated positive effects in reducing the administration of addictive drugs, including nicotine, alcohol, cocaine, and opioids in rodents (Belgers et al., 2016; Chang, Hanania, Mash, & Maillet, 2015). Inspired by the encouraging evidence from pre-clinical studies on animals, attempts to replicate ibogaine synthetically without the cardiac risk and unpleasant side effects are underway. If the evidence continues to show a positive impact on substance use disorders, the addiction treatment world could be revolutionized by breakthroughs with ibogaine-assisted therapies or associated analogs.

IS AN IBOGAINE TRIP NECESSARY TO TREAT SUBSTANCE DEPENDENCY?

In December 2020, a study was published describing a synthetic analog of ibogaine without the cardiac risk and visionary experience (Cameron et al., 2021). The analog showed a reduction in self-administration of alcohol and opioids as well as promising results for depression. Specifically, mice who had been trained to dose themselves with alcohol reduced consumption after a single dose of the ibogaine analog, called TBG. Subsequent studies on TBG and mice showed a complete reversal of stress after a single TBG dose (Lu et al., 2021). Another ibogaine analog, 18-mc, has the same anti-addictive properties but without the risks, unpleasant side effects, and visionary experience. 18-mc is also being studied as an anti-parasitic in Brazil (Delorenzi et al., 2002). However, 18-mc does not modulate neurotrophic factors such as GDNF the way ibogaine does. GDNF is responsible for dopamine survival as well as the increase of neuroplasticity and feelings of well-being that people reference as a protracted benefit of ibogaine. What this will mean for the efficacy of 18-mc months and years later is still unknown.

Analogs such as TBG and 18-mc could change the Western standard treatment model for addiction. In addition, the absence of the visionary experience changes the ibogaine treatment model. These analogs rely on the idea that the dream state is unnecessary for long-lasting recovery, something on which many people are divided.

On the one hand, there is more experience in Gabon over the last 13,000 years than anything we have gathered anecdotally or scientifically in the western practice of ibogaine treatment. The lineage holders of this medicine rely heavily on teachings from the visionary state. Ibogaine providers around the world have seen clients receive life-changing epiphanies during their dream states. Some providers claim that unpleasant side effects are necessary as people who have been using drugs need to learn how to sit with unpleasantness; they see value and healing during this time.

On the other hand, the risks of ibogaine treatment can be high, potentially fatal, and some people are not candidates for it to begin with. Lineage holders of ibogaine have no experience with analogs, making it hard to fully invest in the hypothetical necessity of ibogaine's subjective effects for substance use disorder treatments. Whether the subjective effects or even the use of ibogaine is necessary will remain a topic of high interest in addiction research for the near future.

THE RELATIONSHIP BETWEEN IBOGAINE AND ALCOHOL

Alcohol is a sedative and neurotoxin that negatively affects the brain and body. It is particularly taxing on the brain and liver when used chronically in high doses. In alcohol use disorders, a physical dependence can occur, leading to severe withdrawals that can include medical risks such as seizures or delirium tremens. Due to the risk of seizures, ibogaine should only be given for alcohol dependency once the individual has detoxified from alcohol. Due to the dangers of alcohol withdrawal, this should be done in a medically supervised setting.

Ibogaine modulates and increases the neurotrophic factor GDNF in the brain, reducing cravings and eradicating post-acute withdrawals in alcohol-dependent people. Noribogaine, ibogaine's metabolite, which is long-lasting and has protracted benefits, is theorized to continue to reduce alcohol cravings and also alleviate depression. In a 2005 study that focused on ibogaine's mechanism of action on GDNF and ethanol self-administration in rats, rats showed a dramatic decrease in ethanol intake immediately after ibogaine administration and also two weeks later, suggesting the potential for ibogaine as an effective treatment for alcohol (He et al., 2005). Long-term alcohol use disrupts the brain's ability to produce dopamine and serotonin. There is some evidence that ibogaine can repair these systems (Stanley D. Glick & Maisonneuve, 1998).

Anecdotally, people who have gone to ibogaine treatment centers agree. The introspection and self-reflection that can occur during the dream-like state on ibogaine may also help people who are dependent on alcohol. It may help a person process trauma and events that may contribute to their alcohol use; it may also help a person create a path to move forward (Popik & Skolnick, 1999).

THE RELATIONSHIP BETWEEN IBOGAINE AND COCAINE

Cocaine is a powerful central nervous system stimulant that increases dopamine levels in the brain, resulting in a feeling of euphoria. However, prolonged use of cocaine can lead to changes in brain chemistry, making it difficult for people who use cocaine to feel pleasure without the drug. While the exact mechanism of action is not fully understood, it is believed that ibogaine interacts with serotonin, dopamine, and kappa receptors in the brain, which may play a role in its ability to reduce cravings and withdrawal symptoms, as well as catalyze across NMDA and glutamate neurotransmitters, both thought to be vital for recovery from substance dependency. (Stanley D. Glick & Maisonneuve, 1998).

In an observational study on humans, ibogaine reduced cocaine use as well as elevating mood, alleviating symptoms of depression, and other post-acute withdrawal symptoms, such as low energy. In studies on rodents, after ingesting ibogaine, mice and rats continually decreased their self-administration of cocaine (Sershen, Hashim, & Lajtha, 1994). Among the ibogaine community, many providers and clients talk about a "resetting" process or a complete reset of tolerance from current dependencies. There is some evidence to suggest that neuroadaptation may occur with cocaine and methamphetamine (Alper, 2001).

Ibogaine has shown to be beneficial for the dampening of cravings that arise with cocaine cessation. Noribogaine, ibogaine's long-lasting metabolite, may help alleviate anhedonia and the depression that comes with post-acute withdrawal syndrome (PAWS).

There is scarce research on ibogaine and other stimulants, but one study on ibogaine and methamphetamine suggests that ibogaine works similarly with methamphetamine as it does cocaine. Substances such as cocaine, methamphetamine, amphetamine (Adderall, Vyvanse), and methylphenidate (Ritalin) need to be stopped for a period of time before working with ibogaine.

THE RELATIONSHIP BETWEEN IBOGAINE AND OPIOIDS

Ibogaine has a complex mechanism of action that is not yet fully understood. However, studies show promising results that ibogaine can decrease cravings, prevent relapse for an extended period of time, and lower self-reported feelings of depression (Mash et al., 2000). Both ibogaine and noribogaine bind to mu as well as other opioid receptor sites, although they lack physical responses considered classic of opioids, such as pupil constriction and respiratory depression.

While noribogaine binds as an agonist at mu and kappa opioid receptor sites, it is not a heat-seeking missile: It works across multiple neurotransmitters. Combined effects across systems may be responsible for the interrupting of opioid withdrawals. Ibogaine also has a significant relationship with NMDA receptors (Alper, 2001). This relationship, as well as the modulating of GDNF and BDNF neurotrophic factors, may contribute to the promotion of neuroplasticity and the "reset" feeling many people describe after ibogaine (Marton et al., 2019).

Research on opioid detoxification using ibogaine has primarily focused on heroin and morphine due to the need to be taking short-acting opioids to be a candidate for ibogaine therapy and the prevalence of heroin use disorder. Still, we can reasonably assume persons taking other short-acting opiates, such as oxycodone and hydromorphone, will react similarly to ibogaine. People who use opiates (morphine, heroin) only have to stop their opiate use for 9-12 hours before ibogaine treatment, unlike most other drugs, which require a number of days or weeks. Therefore, abstaining overnight during sleep is enough to proceed. Ibogaine has a profound resetting process with opiates where the individual's tolerance is returned to a pre-dependent state, suggesting neuroadaptive properties. If there is a single substance ibogaine appears to seamlessly be made for, it's short-acting opiates.

The use of long-acting opioid medications and synthetics used in the treatment of OUD, such as methadone, fentanyl, and buprenorphine, disqualify a person from using ibogaine. Persons using these medications or other long-acting opioids will be required to switch to short-acting opioids for successful detoxification and treatment of their OUD. Ibogaine treatment for opiate dependency eliminates nearly all withdrawal symptoms upon the first dosage and also significantly eliminates the possibility of post-acute withdrawal syndrome (PAWS). If PAWS occurs, ibogaine booster doses help eliminate the symptoms.

THE RELATIONSHIP BETWEEN IBOGAINE AND NICOTINE

Nicotine is a highly addictive compound found in tobacco, and smoking is a leading cause of preventable death. Nicotine quickly crosses the blood-brain barrier and agonizes the nicotinic acetylcholine receptor, leading to dopamine release and reinforcement. Once nicotine dependence is established, withdrawal symptoms and cravings from nicotine set in quickly with cessation, increasing stress and cravings. Ibogaine antagonizes Alpha-3-beta-4 receptors and inhibits acetylcholine receptors (S. D. Glick, Maisonneuve, Kitchen, & Fleck, 2002).

Studies have shown ibogaine to be effective for nicotine in dose-dependent amounts in rats (Chang et al., 2015). Rats were shown to reduce nicotine intake by up to 64% with ibogaine. However, the dosage of ibogaine mattered, which means there is a threshold amount of ibogaine that seems to trigger the response necessary for nicotine cessation, and this threshold may be different in different people.

This coincides with anecdotal reports from ibogaine providers who have attempted to treat smokers. It may be worth noting that it is not common for smokers to seek out ibogaine for smoking alone. Usually, smokers have a primary reason for seeking out ibogaine treatment, something they are highly motivated to tackle that leads them to treatment. This may be why, anecdotally, reports from providers regarding nicotine are not as positive as studies have shown. The desire to quit must come first.

THE RELATIONSHIP BETWEEN IBOGAINE AND HEROIN

Heroin (diacetylmorphine) is an opiate initially synthesized in 1874 by C. R. Alder Wright, a chemist in England. The name comes from the German word "heroisch," which means powerful or strong. Opioids like heroin are drugs that stimulate and bind to opioid receptors in the brain, which contribute to regulating how we feel pain and emotions like pleasure. Heroin is made from morphine, which is derived from the poppy plant. It produces sedative effects in the central nervous system, blocks emotional and physical pain, and has cough suppressant and antidiarrheal effects.

Heroin is an addictive drug that is commonly smoked, snorted, or injected. When a person takes heroin, it causes a release of dopamine into the part of the brain where the opioid receptors are located, initially producing feelings of intense euphoria and relaxation (Le Merrer, Becker, Befort, & Kieffer, 2009). Repeated heroin use can lead to dependency, tolerance, and physical or psychological (craving) dependence. Heroin withdrawal is when your body starts to react negatively after the heroin use has stopped.

Heroin withdrawal includes symptoms like dysphoria, depression, anxiety, insomnia, diarrhea, sweating, cold sweats, muscle aches, nausea, and vomiting. The withdrawal symptoms can be so severe that they can lead people to take more heroin as they seek to eliminate the pain and discomfort caused by detoxing from this drug.

FENTANYL AND HEROIN: DOES IBOGAINE WORK THE SAME?

Fentanyl is a synthetic opioid with a higher potency than other opiates. It has a much stronger binding affinity than morphine and is 80-100 times more potent, according to the DEA. Unfortunately, fentanyl has become increasingly common as an adulterant in illicit drugs, with most heroin supplies now laced with it. Fentanyl also turns up in other illicit drugs like ketamine, methamphetamine, and cocaine, and accidental overdoses with fentanyl were almost 12x higher in 2019 than they there were in 2013. While adulteration of drug supplies with fentanyl is worrying in and of itself, there are additional concerns that the use of fentanyl could complicate ibogaine use for OUD.

For example, some ibogaine providers have stressed the need for longer short-acting opiate (SAO) switchover times for fentanyl prior to ibogaine treatment, possibly up to two weeks. This means a period of using morphine or (non-adulterated) heroin prior to the use of ibogaine. Despite fentanyl's short-acting effects after ingestion, it has been observed that a single flood dose may not clear all withdrawals from fentanyl and that fentanyl-dependent people may experience post-acute withdrawals.

IS IT SAFE TO DETOX FROM OPIOIDS WITH IBOGAINE?

Opiate detoxification can be a difficult and dangerous process. Home detoxification of heroin with ibogaine is not safe, and ibogaine detoxification should always be done under the care of professionals at an ibogaine treatment center (Alper, Stajić, & Gill, 2012). Opiate detoxes are particularly taxing, and fatalities, as well as adverse medical events, have occurred.

Ibogaine participants should be in good cardiac health and thoroughly screened by their ibogaine provider for other exclusion criteria. Anyone interested in ibogaine must be screened with an EKG, electrolyte, liver, and full metabolic panel before committing to treatment. In some cases, an echocardiogram, stress test, and/or 24-hour Holter might be necessary. Treatment centers should have robust screening procedures, medical staff, monitoring equipment, and access to emergency medical services for optimal safety.

Persons cannot safely ingest ibogaine while taking long-acting opioids, including those like methadone or buprenorphine. The use of short-acting opiates like heroin or morphine is required for the detoxification of opioids with ibogaine. This is because ibogaine has neuroadaptive properties, and while resetting heroin tolerance, ibogaine simultaneously potentiates opiates (Trujillo & Akil, 1991). For this reason, opiate users need to be in the beginning stages of withdrawal from short-acting opiates when they start their ibogaine treatment.

In the case of an individual who may not meet all inclusion criteria, for example, an intravenous heroin user who doesn't have vein access for emergency fluids or a methadone-dependent individual who has no way to switch to an SAO, providers may need to speak to potential clients about the possibility of using a cumulative and low structured dosing protocol rather than a flood dose.

OPIATE DETOX WITH IBOGAINE

Treatment of ibogaine for opiate detoxification typically begins at the first signs of withdrawal, about 8-12 hours after the last use of a short-acting opiate. Test doses may be administered in the days prior to treatment to gauge sensitivity and cardiac response to ibogaine. Once cardiac function has returned to baseline, a "flood does" is administered. A "flood dose" is an industry term for an amount of ibogaine large enough to saturate receptor sites and eradicate withdrawals while also inducing a psychedelic dream-like state. This effectively allows ibogaine to interrupt the withdrawals from SAOs shortly after ingestion. The dose of ibogaine necessary to adequately alleviate opiate withdrawal and craving may be dependent on the severity of the opiate dependency. High habits of heroin or other opiates may require more ibogaine to feel relief from withdrawal symptoms and cravings than someone else (Alper, Lotsof, Frenken, Luciano, & Bastiaans, 1999). Flood doses begin at 8-12mg/kg of ibogaine, with higher doses thought to carry greater risks.

When ingested, ibogaine is metabolized by the liver and converted into a long-acting metabolite called noribogaine. Noribogaine interacts and shares activity with ibogaine across many areas of the brain, including opioid receptors, and may be responsible for many of ibogaine's long-lasting benefits. Multiple studies on the longer-acting noribogaine suggest that noribogaine may be more active at opioid receptor sites than its parent compound and may also provide anti-anxiety effects (Maillet et al., 2015). Noribogaine increases serotonin and binds to 5-HT receptors. It may also block drug cravings, reduce withdrawal symptoms from heroin and opiate treatment, and prevent relapse.

In multiple observational studies of humans, ibogaine was successful in eliminating opiate withdrawal symptoms. One study looked at acute opioid detoxification in 33 individuals (Alper et al., 1999). Seventy-six percent of the patients had zero opiate withdrawals or cravings at 24 hours and 48 hours after their initial dose of ibogaine, and withdrawals were eliminated within three hours of ingestion. The remainder of the group was a mix of people who had minor withdrawal symptoms that were resolved by the second day or no withdrawals but still had cravings, one person who was determined to be underdosed, and one person who died of cardiopulmonary arrest 19 hours after ingestion.

People detoxing from short-acting opiates like heroin have self-reported complete relief of withdrawal symptoms within 1-3 hours and up to 12-24 hours after ibogaine administration (Alper et al., 1999). Tolerance is reduced, and individuals are returned to a novice, pre-addicted state. For some individuals, residual withdrawal symptoms or post-acute withdrawal symptoms (PAWS) may occur, and booster doses of ibogaine may be used.

In one observational study that included a 12-month follow-up, even the patients who resumed opiate use claimed they had positive ibogaine experiences and received insight into their personal situation (Noller, Frampton, & Yazar-Klosinski, 2018). Some depression symptoms were also alleviated.

It is important to note that the farther a person gets away from their ibogaine treatment, the more likely they are to return to opiates, although a significant percentage report using fewer drugs. Ibogaine alone often does not do the job. Studies that have followed up with participants 12 months after ibogaine treatment found lower total abstinence numbers, 30% in one case (Davis, Barsuglia, Windham-Herman, Lynch, & Polanco, 2017). One study paired ibogaine with psychotherapy, and 12 months later 60% of participants were abstinent from opiates (Schenberg, de Castro Comis, Chaves, & da Silveira, 2014). Integration, psychotherapy, or addiction recovery aftercare should be employed in each person's treatment for sustained success.

CAN IBOGAINE REALLY BE USED TO TREAT VARIOUS SUBSTANCE DEPENDENCIES?

Even though ibogaine is often touted as a cure for substance dependencies, the reality is that it is only a catalyst for change. While many people do experience profound transformations after ibogaine treatment, relapse rates increase the longer someone is away from their initial treatment. This is why it is so important to have a proper aftercare and integration plan in place. Without this support, it can be very difficult to maintain the positive changes that were made during treatment. Ibogaine is not a magic bullet, but it can be an immensely powerful tool for transformation. With the right support, it can help people to create lasting change in their lives.

Ibogaine also carries significant cardiac risks as well as other physical risks. Not everyone is a candidate for ibogaine treatment, and everyone interested should be thoroughly medically screened by their potential ibogaine treatment center. This is not a DIY substance and should always be used under the care of trained professionals. The research surrounding substance use disorder is promising, and anyone interested in ibogaine for addiction should vet their ibogaine center choices thoroughly.

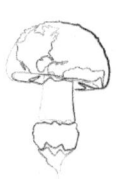

REFERENCES:

- Alper, K. R. (2001). Ibogaine: a review. *Alkaloids Chem Biol, 56*, 1-38. doi:10.1016/s0099-9598(01)56005-8
- Alper, K. R., Lotsof, H. S., Frenken, G. M., Luciano, D. J., & Bastiaans, J. (1999). Treatment of acute opioid withdrawal with ibogaine. *Am J Addict, 8*(3), 234-242. doi:10.1080/105504999305848
- Alper, K. R., Stajić, M., & Gill, J. R. (2012). Fatalities temporally associated with the ingestion of ibogaine. *J Forensic Sci, 57*(2), 398-412. doi:10.1111/j.1556-4029.2011.02008.x
- Belgers, M., Leenaars, M., Homberg, J. R., Ritskes-Hoitinga, M., Schellekens, A. F. A., & Hooijmans, C. R. (2016). Ibogaine and addiction in the animal model, a systematic review and meta-analysis. *Translational psychiatry, 6*(5), e826-e826. doi:10.1038/tp.2016.71

- Cameron, L. P., Tombari, R. J., Lu, J., Pell, A. J., Hurley, Z. Q., Ehinger, Y., . . . Olson, D. E. (2021). A non-hallucinogenic psychedelic analogue with therapeutic potential. *Nature, 589*(7842), 474-479. doi:10.1038/s41586-020-3008-z
- Chang, Q., Hanania, T., Mash, D. C., & Maillet, E. L. (2015). Noribogaine reduces nicotine self-administration in rats. *Journal of psychopharmacology (Oxford, England), 29*(6), 704-711. doi:10.1177/0269881115584461
- Davis, A. K., Barsuglia, J. P., Windham-Herman, A.-M., Lynch, M., & Polanco, M. (2017). Subjective effectiveness of ibogaine treatment for problematic opioid consumption: Short- and long-term outcomes and current psychological functioning. *Journal of Psychedelic Studies, 1*(2), 65-73. doi:10.1556/2054.01.2017.009
- Delorenzi, J. C., Freire-de-Lima, L., Gattass, C. R., de Andrade Costa, D., He, L., Kuehne, M. E., & Saraiva, E. M. (2002). In vitro activities of iboga alkaloid congeners coronaridine and 18-methoxycoronaridine against Leishmania amazonensis. *Antimicrob Agents Chemother, 46*(7), 2111-2115. doi:10.1128/aac.46.7.2111-2115.2002
- Glick, S. D., & Maisonneuve, I. M. (1998). Mechanisms of Antiaddictive Actions of Ibogainea. *Annals of the New York Academy of Sciences, 844*(1), 214-226. doi:https://doi.org/10.1111/j.1749-6632.1998.tb08237.x
- Glick, S. D., Maisonneuve, I. M., Kitchen, B. A., & Fleck, M. W. (2002). Antagonism of alpha 3 beta 4 nicotinic receptors as a strategy to reduce opioid and stimulant self-administration. *Eur J Pharmacol, 438*(1-2), 99-105. doi:10.1016/s0014-2999(02)01284-0
- He, D. Y., McGough, N. N., Ravindranathan, A., Jeanblanc, J., Logrip, M. L., Phamluong, K., . . . Ron, D. (2005). Glial cell line-derived neurotrophic factor mediates the desirable actions of the anti-addiction drug ibogaine against alcohol

- consumption. *J Neurosci, 25*(3), 619-628. doi:10.1523/jneurosci.3959-04.2005
- Le Merrer, J., Becker, J. A. J., Befort, K., & Kieffer, B. L. (2009). Reward processing by the opioid system in the brain. *Physiological reviews, 89*(4), 1379-1412. doi:10.1152/physrev.00005.2009
- Lu, J., Tjia, M., Mullen, B., Cao, B., Lukasiewicz, K., Shah-Morales, S., . . . Zuo, Y. (2021). An analog of psychedelics restores functional neural circuits disrupted by unpredictable stress. *Molecular Psychiatry, 26*(11), 6237-6252. doi:10.1038/s41380-021-01159-1
- Maillet, E. L., Milon, N., Heghinian, M. D., Fishback, J., Schürer, S. C., Garamszegi, N., & Mash, D. C. (2015). Noribogaine is a G-protein biased κ-opioid receptor agonist. *Neuropharmacology, 99*, 675-688. doi:10.1016/j.neuropharm.2015.08.032
- Marton, S., González, B., Rodríguez-Bottero, S., Miquel, E., Martínez-Palma, L., Pazos, M., . . . Carrera, I. (2019). Ibogaine Administration Modifies GDNF and BDNF Expression in Brain Regions Involved in Mesocorticolimbic and Nigral Dopaminergic Circuits. *Frontiers in pharmacology, 10*, 193-193. doi:10.3389/fphar.2019.00193
- Mash, D. C., Kovera, C. A., Pablo, J., Tyndale, R. F., Ervin, F. D., Williams, I. C., . . . Mayor, M. (2000). Ibogaine: complex pharmacokinetics, concerns for safety, and preliminary efficacy measures. *Ann N Y Acad Sci, 914*, 394-401. doi:10.1111/j.1749-6632.2000.tb05213.x
- Noller, G. E., Frampton, C. M., & Yazar-Klosinski, B. (2018). Ibogaine treatment outcomes for opioid dependence from a twelve-month follow-up observational study. *Am J Drug Alcohol Abuse, 44*(1), 37-46. doi:10.1080/00952990.2017.1310218
- Popik, P., & Skolnick, P. (1999). Chapter 3 - Pharmacology of Ibogaine and Ibogaine-Related Alkaloids. *The Alkaloids:*

Chemistry and Biology, 52.
- Schenberg, E. E., de Castro Comis, M. A., Chaves, B. R., & da Silveira, D. X. (2014). Treating drug dependence with the aid of ibogaine: A retrospective study. *Journal of Psychopharmacology, 28*(11), 993-1000. doi:10.1177/0269881114552713
- Sershen, H., Hashim, A., & Lajtha, A. (1994). Ibogaine reduces preference for cocaine consumption in C57BL/6By mice. *Pharmacology Biochemistry and Behavior, 47*(1), 13-19. doi:https://doi.org/10.1016/0091-3057(94)90105-8
- Trujillo, K. A., & Akil, H. (1991). Inhibition of morphine tolerance and dependence by the NMDA receptor antagonist MK-801. *Science, 251*(4989), 85-87. doi:10.1126/science.1824728

PART TEN
DMT AND 5-MEO-DMT

DMT is "the simplest psychedelic" and "exists in all of our bodies and occurs throughout the plant and animal kingdoms. It is a part of the normal makeup of humans and other mammals; marine animals; grasses and peas; toads and frogs; mushrooms and molds; and barks, flowers, and roots."

Rick Strassman

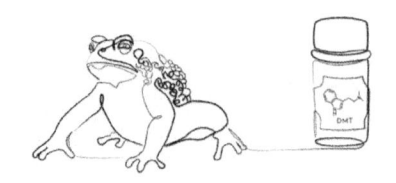

THIRTY-THREE
A BEGINNER'S GUIDE TO DMT
AMBER KRAUS

MEDICALLY REVIEWED BY DR. DAVID COX, PHD, ABPP

Powerful psychedelic drugs like DMT can produce profound experiences, but it's important that you know what you're getting into before you take it. In this beginner's guide to DMT, we will discuss what the drug is, how it works, and the risks involved in taking it. We will also provide some tips for first-time users to have a safe experience.

WHAT IS DMT, AND WHAT ARE ITS EFFECTS ON THE BODY AND MIND?

N,N-Dimethyltryptamine (DMT) is a naturally occurring hallucinogenic tryptamine drug that produces powerful visual and auditory hallucinations. It's an organic chemical found in many plants and, in small amounts, in the nervous systems of mammals. Although scientists are still studying how it occurs in the human brain, some experts believe that endogenous DMT may be produced in the pineal gland and activated in our brains.

DMT is structurally similar to serotonin, a neurotransmitter in the brain that plays a key role in mood and cognition. When ingested, it causes intense changes in perception, leading to an altered state of consciousness that some describe as like a near-death experience.

DMT is thought to bind to serotonin receptors, causing the drug's hallucinogenic effects. DMT is found in several plants native to South America and has been used for centuries by indigenous people for shamanic rituals. When smoked or injected, DMT produces short-lived but incredibly powerful effects.

The DMT experience is often described as a "trip" or "journey." DMT is most often known as an "entheogen," or a substance that may induce divine or spiritual epiphanies. It is the primary psychedelic (although significantly diluted) in Ayahuasca brews. The drug has intense effects that are attractive to DMT users who want a psychedelic experience with a short duration.

EFFECTS

The effects of a DMT trip will be different for every person and may vary from experience to experience. Both the amount and method of ingestion also play a role in the effects of the drug. Generally, the effects of DMT will last for about 15 to 30 minutes.

Physical effects may include:

- Physical euphoria
- Changes in the perception of gravity
- Spatial disorientation
- Sense of separation from the body
- Sense of flying or soaring through space
- Nausea
- Dilated pupils
- Increased heart rate and increased blood pressure
- Seizures (although these are a very rare side effect)

Cognitive effects may include:

- Visual hallucinations
- Auditory hallucinations
- Color enhancement
- Cognitive euphoria
- Mindfulness
- Intense emotions
- Changes in perception of time and reality
- Spiritual insights or epiphanies
- Anxiety
- Delusion
- Memory suppression
- Unity and inter-connectedness
- Perception of eternalism
- Feelings of leaving one's body, similar to those reported in near-death experiences

HISTORY OF DMT

DMT is a highly potent and psychoactive drug found in many plants indigenous to Central and South America, including the ayahuasca vine. It has been used in psychedelic rituals and practices for thousands of years. It is a key ingredient in the psychedelic brew ayahuasca, which is used by shamans and spiritual healers in ceremonies to induce altered states of consciousness.

DMT was first synthesized in the 1930s by Dr. Richard Manske, a German-Canadian chemist. DMT's hallucinogenic properties were not discovered until Hungarian chemist and psychiatrist Dr. Stephen Szara extracted it from the Mimosa hostilis plant and administered it to himself in 1956. Jumping forward, from 1990 to 1995, Dr. Rick Strassman conducted research on 60 volunteers with DMT

(Strassman, 2001). This study became the foundation for his book DMT: The Spirit Molecule, which was also released as a documentary in 2010. Dr. Strassman referred to DMT as the "spirit molecule" because of the similarities to religious and spiritual experiences, including "visions, voices, a seeming separation of consciousness from the body, extreme emotional states, and contact with seemingly discarnate intelligences."

WHAT IS DMT USED FOR TODAY?

In addition to recreational use, DMT is primarily used for spiritual and religious purposes, particularly when brewed with the ayahuasca vine. Some people also use DMT for self-exploration and personal growth. DMT is currently classified as a Schedule 1 drug—a controlled substance that is not legal for recreational use in the United States—but can be used by researchers as long as approval is obtained by the Food and Drug Administration (FDA) and Drug Enforcement Administration (DEA).

DMT is not currently approved for any medical use in the United States. However, it is being studied as a potential treatment for various mental health conditions. In the history of the use of DMT-containing therapeutics, ayahuasca has the most research. A 2016 MRI study conducted by Dr. Rafael G Dos Santos and colleagues on people who have used ayahuasca for long periods of time demonstrated measurable changes in the brain (Dos Santos, Bouso, & Hallak, 2017). A 2007 study by the same professor showed that long-term ayahuasca users had reduced ratings of hopelessness (Santos, Landeira-Fernandez, Strassman, Motta, & Cruz, 2007), while a 2015 study by Dr. Flavia Osorio produced marked improvement in depressive symptoms with no mania or hypomania for up to 21 days following a single dose (Osório Fde et al., 2015).

There are considerable anecdotal reports from people who have taken DMT that it produced profound and positive effects on their mental health. These data suggest evidence for potential antidepressant and antianxiety uses; however, further research is needed to determine the effectiveness. To that end, Yale University is currently sponsoring a dose-escalation open-label study of DMT in humans, where the results will be used for a double-blind, randomized-controlled, crossover study. University Hospital in Basel, Switzerland, has started a double-blind, placebo-controlled study investigating the subjective and involuntary/unconscious effects of DMT in healthy subjects.

Drug and Alcohol Dependence

Substance abuse disorders like drug and alcohol dependence are notorious for being difficult to overcome and are often treatment-resistant. Early clinical trials are exploring the possibility of DMT as a treatment for substance abuse disorders. Trials are exploring the drug's effect on the central nervous system and its subjective effects. Researchers are looking into its potential impact as a therapeutic agent to treat alcohol and drug abuse.

Depression

Depression is a serious mental health condition that can be difficult to treat. There is evidence that DMT may be effective alongside therapy to treat otherwise treatment-resistant depression. In a 2020 Johns Hopkins study led by Alan K Davis and published in the *Journal of Psychopharmacology*, researchers found that "DMT could show promise as an adjunct to therapy for people with mood and behavioral problems" (Davis et al., 2020).

Stroke Recovery

Algernon Pharmaceuticals, a clinical-stage drug development company that focuses specifically on stroke recovery, is currently investigating whether sub-perceptual doses (meaning doses that do not produce any psychedelic effects) of DMT can improve stroke recovery. The company is planning to conduct a Phase 1 clinical trial to test the safety and efficacy of DMT in stroke patients. The primary focus of the Phase 1 study is to "investigate prolonged intravenous infusion of DMT, for durations which have never been clinically studied."

There is an indication that this treatment may be effective in helping patients recover from a stroke, but much more detailed research will need to be done.

HOW IS DMT MADE, AND HOW IS IT USED?

DMT is a molecule found in nature and can also be made synthetically in a lab. It can be extracted from many Central and South American plants like the ayahuasca vine. Synthetic DMT is typically made in powder form.

DMT can be ingested in many ways, but the most common is through smoking. When smoked, DMT reaches the brain very quickly and produces powerful psychedelic effects. It can also be injected intravenously or sometimes snorted. Both smoked and vaporized DMT can produce an intense but short-lived high.

When taken orally, it is not effective unless combined with another substance that metabolizes it. An example of this is when DMT is used in combination with other substances containing a monoamine oxidase inhibitor (MAOI), such as harmaline, to create an ayahuasca brew.

HOW TO USE DMT SAFELY

DMT is not considered to be addictive, and there is no evidence that it leads to dependence. However, more research is needed on this topic, and it is a powerful drug that should not be taken lightly.

It is important to remember that DMT affects each person differently, and the effects can be unpredictable. There is no known safe dosage of DMT, so it is important to start with a low dose and increase gradually if desired.

If you choose to try smoking DMT or ingesting it in another way, consider the following tips:

- DMT can cause you to lose consciousness and become disconnected from reality. Make sure you are in a safe and comfortable setting and have someone with you who can provide support.
- Start with a low dose. DMT is very potent, so it is important to start with a low dose and increase gradually.
- Avoid mixing DMT with other drugs, whether illegal drugs or prescription medications. DMT can have unpredictable effects when combined with other substances, so it is best to avoid mixing it with anything else.
- Be prepared for the experience. It is important to read about DMT and its effects before you try it. This will help you to be prepared for what to expect.

You should not use DMT if:

- you are pregnant or nursing
- you have high blood pressure
- you have a history of mental health problems, including bipolar disorder or schizophrenia

- you are taking any medication that could interact with it
- you have used it previously and experienced any negative effects

WHAT TO EXPECT WHEN YOU TAKE DMT FOR THE FIRST TIME

When you take DMT for the first time, you can expect to experience anything from intense euphoria and hallucinations to feeling a sense of oneness with the universe. Different intensities of DMT concentrations will produce different results, so it is important to start with a low dose, which is typically somewhere between 30-50mg.

The effects of DMT can range from an intense psychedelic experience to a more mellow visual phenomenon (typically seen as colors and geometry). The main characteristic that people report is the feeling of being "one" with themselves or the universe, often described as a spiritual experience.

Some people choose to use DMT in a guided setting, such as with a therapist or shaman. If you are interested in this option, be sure to do your research and find a facilitator who is qualified to guide you through the experience. Remember that DMT is not legal in most countries, so check local laws before trying it.

Some people may feel fear or anxiety during the experience, but it is important to remember that these feelings will eventually subside. It is also important to be aware that DMT can cause you to lose consciousness, so make sure you are in a safe setting with someone who can provide support.

The experience usually lasts around 15-30 minutes, but it can be shorter or longer depending on the person. After the experience, you may feel drained and need some time to relax. It is important to drink plenty of fluids and eat something light during the hours after experiencing a DMT-induced altered state.

RISKS ASSOCIATED WITH USING DMT AND OTHER PSYCHOACTIVE DRUGS

While further research is needed, DMT is considered to be non-addictive and has a low potential for abuse. There is no known lethal dose of the substance, meaning there appears to be no risk of death by overdose. However, this does not mean that it is completely without risk.

Like other psychedelic drugs, DMT can cause users to experience extreme anxiety, paranoia, and fear. In some cases, these effects can be so severe that people may require psychiatric intervention.

Many psychoactive drugs that are considered reasonably safe to use on their own can be dangerous or even life-threatening if combined with other substances. Here is a list of known substances that can have negative side effects when combined with DMT:

- **Lithium:** When taken with lithium, there is anecdotal evidence of significantly increasing the risk of psychosis and seizures.
- **Cannabis:** Using cannabis alongside DMT may cause psychological reactions like anxiety, paranoia, or panic attacks.
- **Cocaine:** When combined with DMT, stimulants like cocaine and amphetamines may result in thought loops, paranoia, mania, or psychosis.
- **Tramadol:** Tramadol lowers the threshold for seizures, which makes it a dangerous combination when used with DMT.

DMT: IS IT FOR YOU?

DMT can be a powerful and life-changing experience, but it's important to remember that it is not completely without risk. Before you decide to try DMT, make sure you are aware of the risks involved and take all necessary safety precautions.

If you do choose to embark on a DMT journey, be prepared for anything—the effects will be different for every person and may vary from trip to trip. Remember, always use caution when experimenting with psychedelics and seek out a safe setting in which to do so. With proper preparation and understanding of the risks involved, DMT can provide profound spiritual experiences that have many benefits.

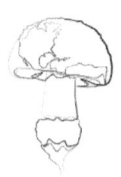

REFERENCES:

- Davis, A. K., Clifton, J. M., Weaver, E. G., Hurwitz, E. S., Johnson, M. W., & Griffiths, R. R. (2020). Survey of entity encounter experiences occasioned by inhaled N,N-dimethyltryptamine: Phenomenology, interpretation, and enduring effects. *Journal of Psychopharmacology, 34*(9), 1008-1020. doi:10.1177/0269881120916143
- Dos Santos, R. G., Bouso, J. C., & Hallak, J. E. C. (2017). Ayahuasca, dimethyltryptamine, and psychosis: a systematic review of human studies. *Ther Adv Psychopharmacol, 7*(4), 141-157. doi:10.1177/2045125316689030
- Osório Fde, L., Sanches, R. F., Macedo, L. R., Santos, R. G., Maia-de-Oliveira, J. P., Wichert-Ana, L., . . . Hallak, J. E. (2015). Antidepressant effects of a single dose of

ayahuasca in patients with recurrent depression: a preliminary report. *Braz J Psychiatry, 37*(1), 13-20. doi:10.1590/1516-4446-2014-1496
- Santos, R. G., Landeira-Fernandez, J., Strassman, R. J., Motta, V., & Cruz, A. P. (2007). Effects of ayahuasca on psychometric measures of anxiety, panic-like and hopelessness in Santo Daime members. *J Ethnopharmacol, 112*(3), 507-513. doi:10.1016/j.jep.2007.04.012
- Strassman, R. (2001). *DMT: The spirit molecule: A doctor's revolutionary research into the biology of near-death and mystical experiences*: Simon and Schuster.

THIRTY-FOUR
A BEGINNER'S GUIDE TO 5-MEO-DMT
AMBER KRAUS

MEDICALLY REVIEWED BY DR. DAVID COX, PHD, ABPP

5-MeO-DMT is a powerful psychedelic compound that has been used for centuries by indigenous cultures all over the world. Today, it is making a comeback as people are beginning to realize the potential therapeutic benefits of this powerful medicine.

WHAT IS 5-MEO-DMT?

5-Methoxy-N,N-dimethyltryptamine (5-MeO-DMT) is found in the venom of the *Bufo alvarius* toad and in certain plants. It has been used for centuries in shamanic rituals and is considered to be one of the most potent psychedelics a human being can ingest.

The earliest documented use of 5-MeO-DMT dates back 3,000 years ago in the form of crushed seeds known as Yopo, which are still utilized in spiritual ceremonies in Venezuela, Colombia, and Brazil. Since then, it has been used by many people seeking a powerful spiritual experience.

5-MeO-DMT is structurally related to DMT and 5-HO-DMT. It is reputed to produce the most powerful and intense psychedelic states of all the psychedelics in the tryptamine class. 5-MeO-DMT shares a similar chemical structure with serotonin, which means it binds to and stimulates serotonin receptors in the central nervous system of our brains, which leads to a psychedelic state.

"TOAD VENOM THAT YOU SMOKE"

If you Google the term "toad venom that you smoke," you'll go deep into a rabbit hole of pop culture icons and celebrities who have "died" and become reborn after their experiences with toad venom. Everyone from Chelsea Handler and Mike Tyson to President Biden's son is talking about how "smoking the toad" has had profound, life-changing, long-term effects.

"Smoking the toad" refers to smoking toad venom that has been excreted and then dried into a paste. The Colorado River Toad secretes a white milky substance from behind its eyes called 'Bufotoxin.' This contains up to 30% 5-MeO-DMT by mass, as well as other substances such as Bufotenine, DMT, NMT, DET, and N-Methylserotonin.

While people like Dr. Ralph Metzner, a former professor at the California Institute of Integral Studies, had been doing field research with 5-MeO-DMT for over 30 years, there has been a recent surge of interest in media and academia. Perhaps due to its recent spike in popularity and increased exposure from celebrities, there's a concern among scientists and researchers that the *Bufo alvarius* may be on a quick road to becoming endangered. Environmentalists are encouraging the psychedelic community to seek out synthesized versions of the drug, which still produce the same effects but without the need to harm the toad species. There is no evidence that the synthetic 5-MeO-DMT is different from the natural version secreted by the *Bufo alvarius* toad.

5-MEO-DMT IS NOT THE SAME AS DMT

It's important to note that 5-MeO-DMT and DMT are NOT the same things. 5-MeO-DMT is structurally similar to DMT, but the two drugs have some important differences. 5-MeO-DMT is active at much lower doses than DMT and has a lower toxicity threshold. 5-MeO-DMT also produces different effects than DMT, with users reporting very intense experiences.

Because of its potent effects, 5-MeO-DMT is not always well tolerated by users, and it can cause anxiety and paranoia. For these reasons, it is important to understand the differences between 5-MeO-DMT and DMT before using either drug.

TODAY'S LEGAL STATUS: 5-MEO-DMT IS A CONTROLLED SUBSTANCE

In the United States, 5-MeO-DMT is currently classified by the Drug Enforcement Administration (DEA) as a Schedule I drug according to the Controlled Substances Act. This means that it is illegal to manufacture, buy, sell, or possess 5-MeO-DMT without a license from the DEA. 5-MeO-DMT is also a controlled substance in many other countries, including Canada and the United Kingdom.

Despite its legal status, it is widely available and is often used for spiritual and therapeutic purposes. It is important to remember that buying 5-MeO-DMT from an unregulated source can be dangerous, as there is no way to know if the product is pure or safe.

HOW 5-MEO-DMT IS USED TODAY

Like many other psychedelic drugs, 5-MeO-DMT is most often used recreationally by people seeking a powerful spiritual experience. It is also used by some therapists as a way to treat mental health disorders such as anxiety and depression; however, this is not legal in the United States.

In a 2018 Johns Hopkins survey of 515 respondents published in the *Journal of Psychopharmacology*, 90% reported moderate-to-strong mystical-type experiences, including awe, amazement, and an experience of pure being/awareness (Alan K. Davis, Barsuglia, Lancelotta, Grant, & Renn, 2018; A. K. Davis, So, Lancelotta, Barsuglia, & Griffiths, 2019). Further, of those who reported being diagnosed with mental health disorders, 79% reported an improvement in depression, 69% with anxiety, 66% with alcoholism, and 60% with drug use disorder.

DOSAGE AND CONSUMPTION

5-MeO-DMT is typically smoked or vaporized, and it produces a short but intense experience that is often described as life-changing. Doses vary depending on whether the drug is produced synthetically or naturally derived. Be careful when measuring the dose of 5-MeO-DMT because it is active in a single dose as small as 3mg. If you are not precise with your measurements, you could accidentally take too much.

The drug produces intense hallucinations and can be dangerous if used improperly, so it is important to be aware of the dose you are taking. Anyone who is new to the drug or to psychedelic experiences should start with a low dose. It is also important to have someone with you who can support you during your experience and provide guidance on dosages, like a qualified shaman or experienced psychedelics user.

Naturally Derived (Toad Venom)

- Small: 10-20 mg
- Medium: 20-40 mg
- Large: 40-60+ mg

Produced Synthetically

- Small: 3-6 mg
- Medium: 6-10 mg
- Large: 11-15+ mg

EFFECTS

5-MeO-DMT is a short-acting psychedelic drug. The duration of the experience is shorter than other more common psychedelics like lysergic acid diethylamide (LSD) or psilocybin.

When vaporized and inhaled, effects begin almost instantaneously. The effects vary depending on the individual, but they typically only last for a short time, around 30-45 minutes. After the effects wear off, users often report feeling refreshed and relaxed.

People often have intense experiences that can be difficult to remember. Some have feelings of a mystical union or feel like they are not separate from their experience. These experiences can also include a transpersonal nature, which means that the person feels like their experience is beyond their individual self.

The entheogenic experience is similar to LSD and psilocybin in terms of psychedelic effects; it can range from uplifting and spiritually significant to devastating and psychologically harmful.

Physical effects may include:

- spontaneous bodily sensations

- physical euphoria
- changes in felt gravity
- muscle contractions or spasms
- motor control loss
- nausea
- pupil dilation
- spatial disorientation

Cognitive effects may include:

- amnesia
- anxiety
- confusion
- emotional enhancement
- memory suppression
- mindfulness
- rejuvenation
- thought connectivity
- ego death
- time distortion

CLINICAL DEVELOPMENT OF 5-MEO-DMT

Although it is not currently approved for medical use, some researchers believe that 5-MeO-DMT has therapeutic potential. It is being studied in early clinical trials as a possible treatment for anxiety and depression, as well as other psychological disorders (Sherwood, Claveau, Lancelotta, Kaylo, & Lenoch, 2020). A 2021 narrative synthesis of research published by Ermakova and colleagues in the *Journal of Psychopharmacology* found over 220 research articles on this powerful substance (Ermakova, Dunbar, Rucker, & Johnson, 2022).

Early studies have shown that 5-MeO-DMT can help treat various mental health conditions, including anxiety, depression, and post-traumatic stress disorder (PTSD). Some research suggests that it may also be effective in treating substance abuse disorders. However, much of the research on 5-MeO-DMT is in its early stages, and more research is needed to confirm its therapeutic potential. Nevertheless, the emerging evidence suggests that 5-MeO-DMT could be a promising new treatment for mental illness.

Researchers at the John Hopkins Center for Psychedelic Research have begun studying 5-MeO-DMT, with researcher Dr. Alan K. Davis believing this drug could effectively treat mental illness due to neurological changes that occur within users' brains after they take it (A. K. Davis et al., 2019).

Anxiety and Depression

5-MeO-DMT has shown promise in the treatment of anxiety and depression, as well as other mental health conditions (Uthaug et al., 2019). A 2019 Johns Hopkins University survey of 362 adults who used 5-MeO-DMT found that 80 percent of participants reported improvements in depression and anxiety after use (A. K. Davis et al., 2019). This survey also showed that 5-MeO-DMT effectively reduced symptoms of anxiety and depression in participants with treatment-resistant depression or other mental illnesses. The study found that 5-MeO-DMT was well tolerated and had a low incidence of adverse effects. Initial research appears to align not just with anecdotal reports but multiple studies on the pharmacological effects in animals, findings from population-based surveys, and findings with related psychoactive tryptamines such as psilocybin for challenges arising from anxiety or depression. Researchers believe that the therapeutic potential of 5-MeO-DMT and other tryptamines appears to be connected with their ability to occasion mystical experiences. The lasting beneficial effects of these mystical experiences have been well documented.

PTSD

PTSD is a condition that can develop after a person experiences a traumatic event. PTSD can cause a range of symptoms, including flashbacks, intrusive thoughts, and extreme anxiety. While PTSD can be treated with medication and therapy, some people find that these treatments are not effective. For these individuals, alternative treatments—such as 5-MeO-DMT—may be worth exploring.

While more research is needed to determine the safety and efficacy of 5-MeO-DMT for PTSD treatment, the potential benefits warrant further investigation. Some people believe that 5-MeO-DMT can help heal the trauma stored in the brain, providing relief from PTSD symptoms.

Substance Abuse

5-MeO-DMT may be beneficial for those who suffer from drug abuse or alcohol abuse because it can help promote ego death, which is the dissolution of the self. This can be helpful for those who are struggling with addiction because it can help them see that their addiction is not who they are. 5-MeO-DMT can also help to reduce cravings and increase self-awareness. For these reasons, 5-MeO-DMT may be an effective treatment for those struggling with substance abuse.

Adjunct to Ibogaine Therapy

For centuries, iboga roots have been used in traditional medicine to promote healing and spiritual growth. In recent years, ibogaine therapy has become increasingly popular as a treatment for patients suffering from addiction and mental health disorders. Now, some researchers are exploring the potential of 5-MeO-DMT as an adjunct to ibogaine therapy because the two substances are structurally similar.

Like ibogaine, it is thought to be capable of resetting the brain's chemistry and helping to break the cycle of addictive behaviors. When used together, ibogaine and 5-MeO-DMT may offer more comprehensive and effective treatment for addiction than either substance alone; however, more research is needed.

TIPS FOR USING 5-MEO-DMT AND OTHER PSYCHOACTIVE DRUGS SAFELY AND RESPONSIBLY

Although most psychedelic drugs are still classified as illegal in the United States and many other countries, many people choose to use these substances for religious or mystical experiences, for a psychedelic experience as an adjunct to therapy, or for the exploration of increased life satisfaction. If you do choose to use any psychedelic drug, there are several things to keep in mind in order to have a safe and positive experience.

Set and Setting

When taking any psychoactive drug, it is important to be aware of the set and setting in which you experience a trip. Set refers to the mindset of the person taking the drug, while setting refers to the physical environment in which the drug is taken. Both set and setting can have a significant impact on the effects of the drug.

For example, someone who is feeling anxious or stressed may have a bad experience if they take 5-MeO-DMT or other psychedelics in an uncontrolled environment. On the other hand, someone who is feeling relaxed and comfortable may have a positive experience. It is important to choose a safe and familiar setting, such as your own home. You should also set an intention for your experience, such as wanting to feel more connected to nature or to explore your own psyche.

5-MeO-DMT can cause people to become incapacitated, so it is important to have someone with you who can keep you safe during and after the trip. Remember that the drug can intensify your surroundings and make it difficult to orient yourself, so you should choose a place that is safe and away from large bodies of water, roads or highways, or other dangerous surroundings.

Toxicity and Harm Potential

The relative absence of research on 5-MeO-DMT limits our understanding of the risks associated with this medicine. Some people have reported feeling anxiety, panic attacks, and disturbed sleep after using 5-MeO-DMT, while a small portion of others found it difficult to integrate unwanted or overpowering realizations or insights. These effects can last for weeks after the experience. Using a low, measured dose can help to avoid unexpected or overwhelming effects.

The Johns Hopkins survey and anecdotal evidence from healthy volunteers suggests that there are unlikely to be any negative health effects attributed to simply trying 5-MeO-DMT by itself at low and moderate doses. That being said, very few respondents of the Johns Hopkins survey reported being diagnosed with previous existing physical medical conditions, so caution is warranted.

Pre-Existing Conditions

People with lung conditions or asthma should avoid smoking 5-MeO-DMT because they are more likely to have adverse effects.

Additionally, people with cardiac problems should avoid using 5-MeO-DMT because it can increase heart rate.

As with other psychedelics, people predisposed to or suffering from schizophrenia or psychosis might experience an onset or worsening of symptoms from 5-MeO-DMT use and should not use this or any other psychedelic substances.

Drug Interactivity

There are a number of drugs that are listed as dangerous to take along with 5-MeO-DMT, including:

- 2C-T-X
- 2C-X
- Cannabis
- DOx
- MDMA
- Mescaline
- NBOMe
- Amphetamines
- Cocaine
- DXM
- Tramadol
- aMT
- MAOIs
- PCP

Potential for Addiction

Animals are commonly used when studying a drug's addiction potential, and there are no published reports on whether laboratory animals choose to self-administer 5-MeO-DMT. There are, however, numerous studies with other classical psychedelics, and, in each case, the laboratory animals either did not self-administer or they did so only occasionally. There is also evidence that the 5-HT_{2c} receptor agonists like those found in 5-MeO-DMT possess anti-addictive properties.

A 2018 human retrospective study by Alan K. Davis from Johns Hopkins and colleagues found that 5-MeO-DMT is not often used recreationally but is more commonly used for spiritual exploration or healing purposes, with 68% of the participants selecting this reason (Alan K. Davis et al., 2018). Only a small number of participants reported using it more than once a year, and the majority indicated that they use a single dose in ceremonial or supportive contexts. Taken together, this suggests that there is a low potential for addiction with 5-MeO-DMT.

If you're looking for a profound, spiritual, psychedelic experience, 5-MeO-DMT might be for you. As one of the most potent psychedelics currently known, it is sure to cause an intense reaction; therefore, it is important to be properly prepared before using 5-MeO-DMT and to have someone with you who can support you during your experience. If you are interested in using 5-MeO-DMT, make sure to do your research and talk to a qualified professional before doing so. 5-MeO-DMT can be a powerful tool for personal growth and healing and, in many cases, can result in sustained enhancement of life satisfaction, but it should not be taken lightly.

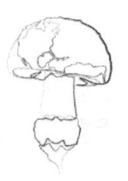

REFERENCES:

- Davis, A. K., Barsuglia, J. P., Lancelotta, R., Grant, R. M., & Renn, E. (2018). The epidemiology of 5-methoxy- N, N-dimethyltryptamine (5-MeO-DMT) use: Benefits, consequences, patterns of use, subjective effects, and reasons for consumption. *Journal of psychopharmacology (Oxford, England), 32*(7), 779-792. doi:10.1177/0269881118769063
- Davis, A. K., So, S., Lancelotta, R., Barsuglia, J. P., & Griffiths, R. R. (2019). 5-methoxy-N,N-dimethyltryptamine (5-MeO-DMT) used in a naturalistic group setting is associated with unintended improvements in depression and anxiety. *Am J Drug Alcohol Abuse, 45*(2), 161-169. doi:10.1080/00952990.2018.1545024
- Ermakova, A. O., Dunbar, F., Rucker, J., & Johnson, M. W. (2022). A narrative synthesis of research with 5-MeO-DMT. *Journal of Psychopharmacology, 36*(3), 273-294. doi:10.1177/02698811211050543
- Sherwood, A. M., Claveau, R., Lancelotta, R., Kaylo, K. W., & Lenoch, K. (2020). Synthesis and Characterization of 5-MeO-DMT Succinate for Clinical Use. *ACS Omega, 5*(49), 32067-32075. doi:10.1021/acsomega.0c05099
- Uthaug, M. V., Lancelotta, R., van Oorsouw, K., Kuypers, K. P. C., Mason, N., Rak, J., . . . Ramaekers, J. G. (2019). A single inhalation of vapor from dried toad secretion containing 5-methoxy-N,N-dimethyltryptamine (5-MeO-DMT) in a naturalistic setting is related to sustained enhancement of satisfaction with life, mindfulness-related capacities, and a decrement of psychopathological symptoms. *Psychopharmacology, 236*(9), 2653-2666. doi:10.1007/s00213-019-05236-w

Printed in Great Britain
by Amazon